The TIME

of my LIFE

---

*...began when the doctor
numbered my days*

Marc McCoy

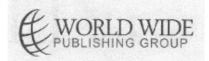

7710-T Cherry Park Drive, Ste 224
Houston, TX 77095
713-766-4271
www.WorldwidePublishingGroup.com

Paperback: 978-0-578-43129-1

Published in the United States of America

Contents

Acknowledgements 5

Chapter 1 - Revelation 7

Chapter 2 - Farewell Tour – Phase One 17

Chapter 3 - The Diagnosis.. 27

Chapter 4 - Acceptance 41

Chapter 5 - Chemotherapy 53

Chapter 6 - Heaven.. 65

Chapter 7 - Farewell Tour – Phase Two 73

Chapter 8 - Preparations for Transplant................................ 83

Chapter 9 - Stem Cell Transplant... 101

Chapter 10 - Post Transplant... 113

Chapter 11 - Early Recovery... 127

Chapter 12 - Mid-Recovery 143

Chapter 13 - Resolutions... 155

Chapter 14 - Next Steps 171

Appendix A - Donor Letters 179

Appendix B - Scriptures on Living for Today 185

Appendix C - Be the Match Info... 195

Appendix D – Critical Decisions 199

So, teach us to number our days,

That we may gain a heart of wisdom.

Psalm 90:12

NKJV

Acknowledgements

She's been by my side for over 40 years. She never left my side when I needed her most. To Cindy, my wife, my best friend, my confidant and now my caregiver who sacrificed so much for me, I love you. Without you, I would have missed The TIME of my LIFE.

I am most grateful to Dr. Steven Kornblau at the MD Anderson Cancer Center in Houston, Texas. His expert care and medical strategies guided me through the most difficult physical challenge of my life.

The nursing team on the 18th floor at the MD Anderson Cancer Hospital is the best of the best. I thank you for putting up with me, and I'm sure I owe an apology or two.

My transplant buddies included Todd, Jim, and Jacob. I thank you for your words of encouragement, putting up with my bad jokes and sharing the grueling experience of a stem cell transplant.

To Todd and Mack, cancer patients who didn't make it, I miss you.

To my friend, Skeeter, who said, "You really ought to write a book," I miss you and pledge to help your family carry on.

To the Walston Group at The Woodlands United Methodist Church, I thank you. You carried me through the transplant, poured over early drafts of this book, provided excellent critiques and helped a novice storyteller become an author.

To the hundreds of believers who prayed fervently for me, please accept my appreciation. Those prayers were powerful, and our healing God answered every one.

To an anonymous stem cell donor on another continent, your gracious gift saved a thankful man's life.

To caregivers the world over, everyone who has endured a medical procedure of any kind owes you a deep debt of gratitude. Please accept our thanks.

To the Almighty God, my savior Jesus Christ and the Holy Spirit that dwells inside me, my praise and gratitude are endless. You provided the strength to endure the physical challenges. You provided peace and comfort. You provided light in so many dark places. You provided the words for this book and the mission to share the benefits of recognizing the short number of our days. You showed me that without a doubt, these past few challenging years had been The TIME of my LIFE.

Chapter 1
The Revelation

November 11, Day -581

Today, I could run forever. I'm giving the pavement a good pounding with my loud red running shoes. The pavement usually pounds back but not today. My strides are long and effortless, my legs feel strong, and my lungs are stretching just enough to handle an extra measure of the fresh morning air. I'll have no trouble keeping up this pace for another 30-minutes and completing my six-mile run in record time. Not too shabby for a guy in his 60's.

Another guy about my age runs past me in the other direction, and we exchange waves. He's running faster, and I wonder if I could push myself a little harder. I don't think so. No, I'll maintain my current pace and hang onto this feeling of strength and accomplishment a little while longer.

The pavement along the Waterway turns to the right, and I notice a tall grey egret in striking position. He's been strolling along the edge of the manmade canal looking for a fish swimming a little too close to the surface. One quick well-trained strike and breakfast was served.

"Hello, Grey!" I shouted. "Not the right one?" I asked as he seemed to return to his normal upright stance.

He answered with a squawk and flew off to find another position. If he doesn't want to talk, no problem. Many other egrets, ducks, and turtles will be happy to chat along the Waterway.

A few minutes down the concrete path a bridge would require paying a little more attention to navigate a couple of sharp turns on the connecting ramp. The canal on my left opened into a lake surrounded by modern office buildings and restaurant patios, and the bridge provided the last chance to cross over. Then, on to the mall, around a few more restaurant patios, past the square with a small park and band shell and on down to the stone waterfalls next to a large wide-open green space. The course stretched out six miles if you ran it twice.

I run this course every other day to stay in shape and clear my mind, but today's run would change me. It would shake me to my core and alter my outlook on nearly everything in my life.

Running lulls me into deep thinking and meditation. No headphones or earbuds for me. If I'm not absorbing the natural beauty of the Waterway, I'll replay some scene from my past, recall a scripture that I had read recently or express praise and appreciation to my Father and Savior. I want the full outdoor experience and the freedom to let my mind wander.

Deep thinking and meditation include short prayers on various subjects. Free flowing meditation shifts to a specific prayer then back to deep contemplation of a different notion. It's an enjoyable time at the feet of the Father taking comfort just being in His presence. I speak freely with Him sharing my thoughts and issues knowing He is already fully aware of each one. He responds with a subtle suggestion or a feeling that I am going in the right direction. Often, I'll sense His conviction and the need to shift gears to come into alignment with His perfect plan. Sometimes it's a gentle nudge. Or, it could be a sharper rebuke and a command to do something different. Either way, if you listen and obey, the feeling of joy afterward is unmatched by anything else.

A subtle suggestion came first. Stop running, stop talking and listen. I had every intention of doing that after completing the six miles and celebrating the record pace. Once I finished the run, I'd find a quiet place to sit, cool down, open my ears and give Him my full attention. The suggestion was amplified into a stronger nudge with more specific instructions to stop immediately and focus my attention on Him. I started looking for a bench or someplace to sit. The nudge escalated to a firm and direct order that wouldn't stand for any more delays.

Stop! Now!

I had received many suggestions and firm nudges over the past few years and was getting better at recognizing and reacting to them. I have even learned to listen actively for convictions from the Holy Spirit if I'm moving in an iffy direction. Direct orders come much less frequently and should not be dismissed. You better stop and listen.

What was the message? What was so important? Why did I have to stop and listen exactly at this moment?

The closest bench called from the front of a Japanese restaurant in Waterway Square. The bench didn't budge even under the full weight of a tired runner. I sat leaning forward with my arms on my thighs catching my breath. I closed my eyes and tried to block out the sound of heavy breathing, delivery trucks, and honking horns. This time of the morning, delivery crews and workers getting their shops ready for the day outnumbered pedestrians and customers. They didn't even notice the guy sitting on the bench with his head bowed and eyes closed.

After a few minutes, the words came. They were soft but firm and resonated from the very back of my mind. They cut right through the noisy traffic of this commercial section of the Waterway.

"I'm calling you home soon."

Simple, brief and to the point. It was not an emotional statement. It was a factual directive meant to be taken at face value. There was no doubt of the meaning of the message, the authority of the message or the source of the message. God told me my days were numbered.

No further explanation was given or necessary. The message stood on its own. I remained in that quiet space for a few minutes with no reaction at all as that direct connection to the Heavenly Father tapered then disappeared. I'm not sure how long I sat on the bench, but I hung on to the connection as long as I could. An atmosphere of peace and certainty surrounded that message, and I didn't want to let it go knowing that I'd then have to deal with it.

But there it went. And, there I sat stunned and numbed with the challenge of getting my arms around it. That was part of the process. Here's the message, now deal with it. Figure it out. Search for the meaning and seek out the proper response. Fortunately, God left me with a good measure of peace and the feeling that I wasn't on my own. He would be right there with me as I sorted things out.

How do you sort out the end of your days? How do you process that? Why do I have to deal with that?

I had many more questions than answers.

Why was He calling me home? Why was He telling me ahead of time? How was my life going to end? What would come of my home, wife, and family? What about all the unfinished business, uncompleted projects and unmet obligations? The quiet space had become a torrent of questions spinning rapidly in and out of my mind. Some doubt crept in. Did I hear what I thought I heard? Did I have the message right? Did I interpret it correctly? Was I taking it too seriously? No chance. It was clear, it was complete, and the message was final.

I struggled under the crushing weight of the revelation. No other thought, notion or idea could penetrate this new reality. The questions began to sort themselves giving way to those with the highest priority. What does "soon" mean? That question topped them all. Peter told us that a day is like a thousand years to the Lord. That's a big spread for a mere mortal trying to decipher how much time he had left. What exactly is the definition of soon?

I struggled mightily with the idea of being a short-timer, but I took some solace in the fact that I was being called home and not someplace else. Home had to be Heaven, right? The gift of salvation I accepted from Jesus Christ, my savior ensured that I would walk through the pearly gates and spend eternity in the place He prepared for me. That fact alone gave me some deep comfort. I never questioned my salvation or the promise of eternal life but hearing it directly from God rendered complete assurance. I needed that.

Clinging to that comfort, I allowed the more practical and distressing questions to swim to the surface. How would I meet my demise? Would I have a traffic accident? Would I contract a fatal illness? Would lightning strike me? None of those questions would be answered but stayed right at the top of my consciousness. Frozen in my spot on the bench, I had no desire to move for fear I'd suffer a fatal fall or get hit by a car crossing the street. I couldn't sit there forever, though, and I knew I had to get going and make my way home. Maybe the term "soon" meant more than a few short minutes. I looked both ways, twice, before gathering the courage to cross the street. I took extra care not to trip on anything and tumble into the Waterway. I made sure I didn't gulp the water too quickly at the drinking fountain. All the regular movements I took for granted were now suspect as each could result in tragedy. I was no longer at home in familiar and safe surroundings. I was a visitor tip-toeing around a series of potential disasters that only I could see.

Minutes turned into hours raising the possibility that I might have a few days left. Maybe even a month or two. I could only hope. Could I hope for enough time to tie up some loose ends?

I retired from a long career in media and marketing a few months ago. I'm still in vacation mode after jumping out of the working world enjoying every moment of not being accountable for something to someone. I filled my time with all those things I never had time to do before and finally exercised the way that I should. Some personal business needed attention like settling my mother's modest estate and looking for my official retirement home which would look and feel something like Margaritaville. I had always envisioned spending my retirement years dressed in a Hawaiian shirt and a pair of flip-flops walking distance from a marina. That vision had now dissolved as there would be no retirement for me. I could let go of mine, but my wife had many years ahead of her. Sadly, I shifted my focus to setting up her retirement without me.

Of all those questions and loose ends spinning around in my head, the thought of abandoning my wife of 42-years haunted me the most. While I wondered what would become of her, God assured that she had a secure place in the palm of His loving hand. She would be fine.

There were many other smaller day-to-day issues that would typically take up much of my attention and concern, but they would surely work themselves out without me. I would set those aside for now.

Surviving to the end of the day felt like a major accomplishment. My mind continued to spin, but my body was tiring and going through the motions doing what it would usually do. I acted out the nightly ritual of preparing for bed. Change into a loose-fitting t-shirt. Turn down the bed. Turn on the TV in the bedroom. Floss. Brush. Wash. Crawl in next to Cindy. Flip through the channels looking for something to watch. I settled on Fixer Upper, but it didn't make any difference. My mind occupied a different world floating through a series of random thoughts all related to the end of my days. And, now, here comes another new fear. The fear of not waking up. Would I die in my sleep? I was afraid to close my eyes, but I couldn't hold them open any longer.

November 12, Day -580

The sun rose right on schedule. When my eyes opened, I felt nothing but gratitude. I was grateful to be alive, stretching next to Cindy in a room full of bright sunlight just like any other day. And what a relief. A few hours of sleep had calmed last night's turbulence. The flood of random thoughts had not yet made its way to the top of my mind. I lingered in the grogginess that was keeping those thoughts from surfacing wanting to keep them away and enjoy this moment as long as I could.

God gave me another day, and I spent most of it in prayer. Whether walking, sitting or eating, I stayed in prayer and continually felt God's presence and His full knowledge of what I was processing and feeling. Do I dare approach Him and seek some clarification? Maybe discuss the terms of His revelation? He allowed me to ask for some time to work out some of the essential but unresolved issues. He knew what was on my mind and agreed to allow enough time to finalize my mother's estate, get my affairs in order and get my wife settled in a new home. I had gone to the Father with a request and received more of His grace. Those projects would take about 90 days to complete when you figured in a preplanned Christmas vacation to visit our daughter's family in Southern California. That vacation would now include a secret house-hunting trip since my wife's version of Margaritaville would undoubtedly include proximity to our four grandchildren.

After spending so much time thinking I could pass away at any moment, a couple of month's breathing room offered some relief. And that begs the question. What to do with the short time remaining? If you were certain you had but three months to live, what would you do with those three months? How would you spend your time? What would be important? What would no longer be of any concern? How would your relationships change?

My wife knew nothing of the revelation. I knew I would tell her at some point, but it didn't seem right at this moment. If I struggled with this weighty new reality how would she deal with it? I plodded through a typical day, and life went on as normal. Or, as normal as it could be for someone carrying the burden of a big secret. I tried desperately to be normal. I made every effort to act as if nothing had changed.

Not telling my wife about the revelation was a type of torture I could hardly bear. Cindy radiated beauty in every way. As attractive as she is on the outside, she is even more stunning on the inside. She is kind and generous to a fault. If she passed by someone who looked confused, Cindy would engage immediately and try to help. If a person dropped their keys, she would be the first to pick them up. If a stranger couldn't find her car in the parking lot, Cindy would drop everything and take up the cause of locating the missing vehicle.

Cindy is also a worrier. In almost every situation, she would contemplate the worst-case scenario and all the other possible adverse outcomes. She would find relief in the fact that outcomes usually wouldn't be as bad as they could have been. The revelation, however, might be too much. The revelation would far exceed any worry she ever had to bear.

I adore this woman. We share everything. Nothing in my life escaped her knowledge. Over our decades together our separate lives had evolved into one life. A transparent, trusting and interdependent life. We had become confidants, soul mates, and best friends.

How do you keep something as impactful as the revelation from someone so precious? Was that even possible? Because I was a horrible poker player and had no skill in keeping secrets, the only course of action was to avoid any conversation even close to the revelation and try to act as normal as possible.

Normal for me now was engulfed by the thought that time was short. The clock was ticking. And, how does one come to terms with that?

For me, it started with a struggle. Every time I experienced something, I was haunted by the thought that it may be the last one of its kind. And, I wrestled with the question of how the end would come. I couldn't shake that notion or even suppress it. It nagged and persisted always looming somewhere in my imagination.

I had to get my arms around this new normal. There were simply no other options.

Fortunately, I had to complete those looming projects. There were things to do, obstacles to overcome, and tasks to accomplish. God graciously provided some time to get those things done, but He didn't give me time to mess around or drag my feet.

Chapter 2
Farewell Tour – Phase One

The retirement phase of my life had taken a sudden and dramatic turn. I had retired early compared to other friends and family members. Days and years ahead were to be spent in good health, downshifted to a lower gear and in a vacation state of mind. Life got in the way and now things would be radically different.

Retirement isn't something I had prepared for or spent a great deal of time planning. I just got tired of working. I managed radio stations for a living and had a passion for turning average performing stations into high performing stations. I enjoyed discovering an unserved audience and developing the programming to attract those listeners. I specialized in the news/talk format and helping AM radio stations compete in an FM world. I had some success as a consultant and advisor, but my real strength was roll up the sleeves, hands-on management. The biggest thrill came from building a large audience with heartfelt community service and accurate local information. I enjoyed the applause, awards, and recognition acquired from those successes. The paychecks weren't bad, either. The exhilaration and the feeling of accomplishment began to fade, however, and no longer justified the grief and grunge work that went with it. I grew weary of the deadlines and drama and annoyed by the purported crisis lurking around every corner.

The last ten years of my career had also been years of personal and spiritual transformation. God was knocking at my door, and I was finally listening. He was convicting me of the intense amount of pride I was harboring. I was being directed to let go of my selfishness, to focus on Him and to seek more godliness. It started with a small step here and another there, but the transformation pace had shifted to a higher gear. While my desire to win in business was waning, my desire to serve my God and mature spiritually was increasing.

I could see the ships moving closer and closer and knew they were on a collision course yet did nothing to stop the crash. After 45 years, I had reached a point where managing radio stations had become more of a job than a passion and a brief stint as Vice President of Marketing for a local home building and home improvement complex didn't turn out to be the ground floor opportunity that I had hoped. Instead of looking for new employment, I went to see my financial advisor with the crazy idea of not working at all. He suggested if I watched my pennies, downsized my lifestyle and got a few lucky breaks along the way, I could pull it off.

A few thoughtful conversations later, Cindy and I gave each other a reassuring look, clasped hands and took the leap. Our permanent vacation and earnest search for Margaritaville began. Exercise, church activities, precious time with Cindy, contemplating tropical retirement locations and all those things I like to do but never had the time to do replaced the time I would usually devote to work. I loved every minute of it and kept my eyes open for volunteer projects or ways I could be helpful to others. That was about six months before the revelation.

The revelation stopped me in my tracks. The revelation cut short that vacation attitude and refocused my priorities. I couldn't focus on myself. I wouldn't be around long. I couldn't focus on the future. There wouldn't be a future. My focus had to be on this moment. I had nothing beyond today. I had to get my arms around a strange new to-do list and a crazy new moment to moment world.

As my world turned itself upside down, my bizarre and sometimes morbid sense of humor remained intact. Leave it to me to see the irony or humor in almost any situation no matter how unusual or bleak it may be.

It is through the lens colored by that bizarre sense of humor that I labeled the next few months "The Farewell Tour," the process of saying goodbye to the people I might not see again and the experiences I may never repeat. It was coming to terms with the temporary nature of everything in this new world.

The Farewell Tour helped me transition out of any "woe is me" attitude I harbored and into acceptance of my circumstances. This phase I kept to myself, and I viewed each event, conversation or experience as potentially my last.

Every six-mile run could be the last. Every time I saw an eagle in flight, it could be the last time I would have that experience. Every time I spoke with someone, it could be the final conversation. That realization changes the perspective and the lens through which you look at every aspect of life.

What do you say in your last conversation with someone? Do you drive past the eagle's nest or do you stop and wait for the babies to pop up and peek out? Do you poke along at a jogger's pace or do you push yourself in what could be the final run? Do you rush through your favorite dessert or do you slow down and savor each bite? Every common event became unique and remarkable. I saw them through new eyes. I felt them at a much deeper level. I cherished them much more. I could feel layers of age and rust lifting from my heart.

Major holidays had a fresh new look. The Halloween and Thanksgiving holidays came and went, and I was sure that they would be my last. Still, I had the peace and comfort of knowing that I had experienced more than my share of pleasant holidays over the years. Christmas was right around the corner, however, and that was a whole new ball game.

Cindy and I were invited to spend Christmas Eve at my daughter's home and experience the event that was Christmas morning with her family. It would have been a "once in a lifetime" event anyway, but there was no question about that now. There would never be another. I couldn't help but look past all the hugs and fun and dread the end of our visit. I would usually get a little emotional at those kinds of goodbyes and was afraid that on this trip I would completely fall apart when it was time to leave. Could I muster the inner strength to say goodbye to them forever?

The grandkids were top priority, but I had some business to attend to as well. I wanted to find a new home somewhere close to their Southern California residence so that Cindy could live nearby. We had discussed the possibility of living closer to the grandchildren many times, and I knew her well enough to assume that's where she would want to be if I were out of the picture. My gracious Father gave me this trip to find that home and oversee the move, but I couldn't count on any more time after the completion of those projects. I packed a strong sense of urgency along with my winter sweaters to make some headway on this project while we were in California.

I adore these grandchildren. It's an emotion somewhere beyond love. The Song of Solomon cannot adequately describe the love I have for them. The greatest poetry ever written falls hopelessly short. Take the strongest and most profound love you have ever felt. Multiply that a thousandfold, and you're almost there. It's that bad. It goes that deep.

After more than a decade of our empty nest phase, our first grandchild made her appearance in 2006. Cindy and I traveled to Arizona for the big event and were able to help bring this bundle of joy home. After about a year, the family moved from Arizona to

Texas and settled about a half hour's drive north of us. It was a dream come true. This gift from God, this beautiful creature was living a few short miles down the freeway. She quickly stole my heart, and all I wanted to do in life was to be a good grandfather. I wanted to show her the world and guide her through life's ups and downs. I wanted to teach her how to ride a bike and warn her about boys. I wanted to be the cool grandpa that she could come to with any problem or celebration.

Most of our free time was devoted to this new family in some way. Whether raking Magnolia leaves in their front yard or attending birthday parties, Cindy and I were of one mind. We wanted to be there and experience every significant event in this child's life. And, her sister's life as it turned out. Our second grandchild entered the world a year later and effortlessly stole my heart yet again.

Imagine the heartbreak when my daughter announced that she would be moving to Southern California. It wasn't merely a bad break; it was devastating. I've received my share of bad news and difficult announcements over the years, but this one took my tender stolen heart and ripped it to pieces. It took months for us to even begin to deal with the concept of separation. I can't say I'm entirely over it to this day. But, that's the way it was. We were no longer a part of their day-to-day life. The move forcefully crushed all our grandparent's dreams. If we were to see them, it would have to be two or three times a year and only a few days at a time. The Christmas vacation was one of these visits that were way too few and much too far between.

With the Christmas visit looming, would this be the right time to tell Cindy about the revelation? Could I come up with the right words? How would she react? Could she process this kind of bombshell and enjoy a major holiday at the same time? I decided that the revelation would ruin what would usually be a joyous occasion. There would be a better time. I would postpone that news and keep the revelation to myself.

December 24, Day -538

We had made more than a dozen trips to Southern California over the past few years trying to spend quality time with the kids and a few days to ourselves attending concerts, sailing or cruising along the coastline north of San Diego. This vacation started in a perfectly normal way. Travel went smoothly, the weather was perfect, and the grandkids were happy to see us. While I knew my time was short, they had no idea. Bicycle rides took place as they usually would. The girls always looked forward to splashing in the hotel pool, and they weren't disappointed this visit. We spend one full day with each of them individually to properly spoil them and give them our full and undivided attention. They decide what they would like to do and we make it happen. Then we toss in a surprise and a new experience they might enjoy.

I try to arrange a surprise for the whole family as well each time we visit, and I made plans for a sailing adventure and whale watching excursion on the USS Hornblower. Thousands of gray whales migrated each winter from their feeding grounds off the coast of Alaska to mating and breeding lagoons in Mexico. Lucky observers on boats in San Diego Bay can watch passing whales spout, see their backs rise out of the water and their tail flukes as they dive back down. The day couldn't be any more perfect with sunny skies and a steady breeze causing a modest chop on the water. The 90-foot Hornblower would easily slice through the waves, so what could go wrong?

Most of the family got seasick and spent much of the sailing adventure close to the trash cans. Madilyn and I had strong stomachs and good sea legs and spent most of the San Diego Bay cruise on the bow of the ship spotting a dozen whales or more.

"Look, Papa. I see it, Papa. Over there!" Madi would say when she saw the whale's spout blow from the surface of the water.

We shouted our approval as the whale's back appeared and its tail came up out of the water. I held her close to protect her from the chilly sea breeze and gave her a little extra squeeze when we saw a whale or a pod of dolphins swimming alongside the boat. It was undoubtedly among my top 10 best grandparenting moments. I knew how rare and extraordinary this experience was and I had to make an extra effort to focus on the joy of the moment rather than the fact that this would be the last experience of its kind. Madi and I shared a great seafaring adventure. The others, not so much. They are still expressing their displeasure at my choice of entertainment venues.

The best part of this trip was the opportunity to experience Christmas Eve and Christmas morning through the eyes of these beautiful young souls. It was truly a Christmas to remember. I savored every moment of this holiday visit in a way I hadn't experienced before. No moment was trivial. There would be no more like them. I was sure of that.

It took every ounce of inner strength to compose myself when it was time to leave. I had thoroughly enjoyed every second of the visit but dreaded this moment. The heart-wrenching goodbye. I moved through it quickly and methodically not wanting to create an emotional spectacle. Each girl got a little extra hug as I let them know again how much I loved them. As we drove away, the girls waved goodbye with the expectation that we would return in a few months to repeat the experience. I waved goodbye for the last time.

Acquiring the ability to savor those extraordinary moments is probably the most valuable lesson learned on The Farewell Tour. Normal busy working lives require us to rush past them or dismiss them as one of many with more to come. We miss most of the best experiences that life has to offer. As painful as suffering through the goodbye was, it is that kind of deeply felt emotion that makes life so special. If only we could shift into a lower gear and live a slower paced life. A life where we believed our time was short and we took the time to enjoy these moments fully. I found it to be a great way to live and only regret that it took a revelation to see it. I consider it to be a great gift that I was able to live at least some of my life that way.

January 24, Day -507

Cindy and I were members of Lakewood Church in Houston before moving 40 miles north to The Woodlands. While we loved our new church home, we missed the impact and grandeur of a Lakewood service.

Lakewood Church is home to Pastor Joel Osteen and is one of Houston's "mega" churches with 43,000 members. A crowd of 10,000 or more pack a typical Sunday morning service to dance, sing and praise their God. Don't let a trip to Houston go by without a visit to Lakewood Church. We needed that powerful experience again and made the one-hour drive south.

On this Sunday, you could sense God's presence. You could feel the music as the band played a medley of our favorite hymns and contemporary Christian songs. Believers danced in front of their seats with arms held high and hands waving to the Heavens. It was a joyous moment when I thought, *"I'm really going to miss this."* And it was at that exact moment when I heard that voice again. Despite the thundering of the music and the activity all around us, I heard that soft voice clearly and distinctly.

"No, you're not."

Another revelation. While I thought this moment was about as good as it could get, that soft voice that packed so much power rattled my bones once again, challenged my feelings and forced me to think about where I was going. It gave me some comfort and excitement knowing that my next move would blow the doors off of this place. An energetic Lakewood service couldn't even compare to the splendor and glory of my Heavenly destination. I couldn't help but smile and hold tightly to those three words spoken so succinctly and impactfully. That simple phrase shook me out of my backward-looking Farewell Tour attitude and pushed me forward to find out more about the future and the resting place a short distance ahead. What would I see in Heaven? What would I do when I arrived? How do I prepare for the trip?

Though not quite as dramatic, there were many other events over the next few months that had a similar impact. They taught me to let go of the things of this world and view their beauty with awe and wonder from a distance. They taught me to turn loose those things that are not so pleasant or a waste of time. The lessons learned during this first phase of The Farewell Tour enhanced my life in many ways.

As the first few months of the year passed, I had completed most of my projects. Loose ends were nailed down. I settled my mother's estate. The California trip didn't result in a new home, but I felt confident that I had set the stage if Cindy wanted to make that move on her own. God had fulfilled His promise, granted me the time and provided the guidance to complete these projects. It's been several months since the revelation.

Now what? When would I be passing on? Tomorrow? Next week? Ten years from now? And, what do I do in the meantime? What was my mission? Was there something I was supposed to accomplish in the time I had remaining?

There was only one thing I knew for sure. I should devote every possible moment to reading the scriptures and learning as much as I could about my Father above and my Savior within. Reading other books seemed pointless. The only thing that seemed to matter was maturing as a Christian. I needed to grow as much as I could before meeting my Creator face-to-face.

The relationships I had with my family and friends became a top priority. I began to care less and less about this world and more and more about my new home in Heaven. After all, this world was passing away quickly. The afterlife was staring me right in the face. I felt God's presence and His message was clear. Stay the course and await further instructions.

God had seen me through the "woe is me" phase and the process of separating myself from this world. He taught me to look ahead to the next world and cast aside the sad thought that each event would be the last and focus on the joy present in each moment. He skillfully chipped away years of age, rust and scars from my aging eyes allowing me to see His creation with more of a childlike sense of wonder.

And, another twist in the road was ahead. The next phase of this journey was lurking around the corner, and it packed a punch I couldn't see coming.

Chapter 3
The Diagnosis

Life in the New Year plodded ahead as normally as it could. I maintained an ambitious running and exercise schedule, and I signed up for every church class and Bible study I could attend. What could be more important than a more in-depth knowledge of God at this phase of my life?

Before the revelation, I filled my new and wide-open schedule with medical checkups and all the procedures that a man over 50 should have. I always felt healthy and vital and saw no need to see a doctor or bother with physical exams over the last 20 years. I deliberately kicked the prostate cancer and other "maintenance" exams down the road. But now, there was no need to put those things off any longer. I had plenty of time to schedule them. No more excuses. Just get them done.

An executive health program at a nearby clinic seemed to be a good option since they offered a complete physical and all the related tests in one day with many results the same day. These results would undoubtedly prove how healthy I was and justify postponing annual physicals for so long. But, once those tests were up to date, I vowed to maintain a regular schedule of all recommended physical exams, checkups and procedures.

I was right about one thing. The physical exam showed that I was in excellent health. The heart, lungs, urinalysis and blood tests all showed normal or better than normal results. All the running I had done paid off on the treadmill. As the doctor was reviewing the print out, he glanced up over his glasses.

"Are you a runner?" He asked.

I nodded affirmatively with a confident smile thinking *"This is going pretty good."*

There was one small problem. It showed up in the blood test. The white blood cell count was below normal. Well below normal. The reading was low enough for them to take another blood sample to see if there was some mistake. That was enough to wipe that overconfident smile off my face and give rise to some genuine concern. Unfortunately, there was no mistake. The second blood test was taken about 90 minutes after the first one and showed the same result: a white blood cell count significantly below normal.

Since I had no recent history of physical exams or blood tests, there was no way for the doctor to look at the results over time to see if that low white blood cell count was in my normal range. Had I maintained a regular schedule of annual exams, there would have been information on hand to make an immediate determination. So much for justifying my medical procrastination. Since the doctors were starting from scratch, they sent me to the clinic's hematology department for a more detailed look at my blood. I had no reason to believe this was anything but a routine follow-up to rule out any problems with the low white blood cell count. Common medications would be prescribed to bring the blood cell counts back to normal, right? Maybe a change in diet? Maybe something to keep a sharp eye on? The hematology department was in a different building a few miles away and shared clinic space with the oncology department. I assured my observant wife that it was merely a coincidence and we shouldn't be alarmed by that.

After a more detailed look at my blood, the recommendation was, of course, more blood tests. The doctor wanted to watch the readings over a more extended period. We dutifully reported for monthly blood tests which were stable for the first five months. When the red blood cells and platelets took a nose dive, the doctor suggested a bone marrow biopsy to see what was going on. Either the stem cells that produce white blood cells weren't doing their job, or something was killing the healthy cells once they matured. A look at my bone marrow would provide more information and required inserting a big needle into my hip bone and extracting the fluid and tissue. It feels about as good as it sounds.

After watching the procedure online, I concluded that the whole biopsy thing was drastic and unnecessary, but it would certainly rule out anything serious since I had no symptoms or felt badly in any way. I finally agreed, but since I had been training for a half marathon, I insisted that the doctor postpone the procedure until after an upcoming race.

A 10k, a little over six miles, was a piece of cake. That distance was routine for me, but a 13.1-mile half marathon was a stretch and required some additional preparation. I pushed the usual 20 miles a week to running over 30 miles a week including one long 13 miler. The half marathon run would take a little over two hours to complete, and I wanted to make sure I could run that length of time at a respectable pace. No stopping and no walking! I had no idea how a bone marrow biopsy would feel and how my body would react, so I stuck to my guns. I overruled the objections of Cindy and the doctor and postponed the procedure to the week after the scheduled race. After all, it could be the last time I ever ran that kind of race at that distance.

With a great sense of accomplishment, I applied an oval 13.1 sticker to the rear window of my car. I not only completed the 13.1-mile race, but I was also telling the world that I was a card-carrying sticker displaying runner. My time wasn't bad, but I had to drag my left leg through the last five miles after pulling a muscle in my calf. Otherwise, my legs were strong, my lungs were healthy, and I outran half the runners in my age group. After a day or two of rest, I even considered running a full marathon. If I could run for a little over two hours, could I run for four or five hours? It would require more training but why not? I had no health symptoms I could attribute to a low white blood cell count. I had no symptoms at all other than the aches and pains that came with the running and exercise.

If I could even consider running a marathon, then how bad could a bone marrow biopsy be? Back in the real world, the day of the procedure is closing in, and there was no way I'd get away with postponing it again. I had to do it. We had to know. Something was eating at my healthy white blood cells.

It turns out; my white blood cells weren't all that healthy. The clinic wouldn't release the biopsy results until I spoke with the hematologist who couldn't see me for another ten days. Cindy is sensing something seriously wrong, but my optimistic logic told me that if it were urgent, they wouldn't delay an appointment for ten days. They would want to see me right away. My skeptical wife wasn't buying it. Her intuition was telling her something was wrong. Seriously wrong.

March 23, Day -448

The appointment day finally came, and we drove to the hematology office speculating on what the results might be. I remained convinced that if it were serious, we would have been given that news earlier. Cindy still had a bad feeling about the diagnosis. She had been doing way too much research online and was fearful of lymphoma or leukemia often associated with a low white blood cell count. Since I still had no symptoms of anything wrong and felt good that morning, I was sure I'd be the one with the correct outcome. I'm glad I didn't make a bet or put any money on it.

We were finally called back to the exam room, and the doctor didn't look happy. She seemed downright distressed and for a good reason. She had to deliver some bad news. She had to convey the results of my bone marrow biopsy which were consistent with a rare disease called Myelodysplastic Syndrome or MDS. She said my bone marrow was producing lousy stem cells that weren't maturing into normal white and red blood cells like they were supposed to. The mutant stem cells are called blasts and measured as a percentage of all the cells. She said my blast count was 16% meaning that 16% of all my stem cells were defective. At the 20% level, the diagnosis changes to Acute Myeloid Leukemia. Good news. I didn't have AML. Then came the bad news. This stage of MDS would typically progress into Acute Myeloid Leukemia in a year or so. Then the doctor used the C word. MDS was bone marrow cancer. Cancer for which there is no cure. Cancer which normally progressed into leukemia. Terminal cancer that would take my life.

Tears are streaming down Cindy's face as the doctor continued with her explanation of MDS and the prognosis. She used a table of numbers printed on a sheet of paper to explain the various outcomes with and without treatment. Sitting right across from the doctor, I could see the table and was reading the upside-down numbers before she could verbalize them. At the stage of MDS I had, the prognosis without treatment was a life expectancy of 1.1 years. She tried to move past that number to some of the other possible outcomes.

I rudely interrupted the presentation. "Hey, wait a minute, here. Am I reading this right? That without treatment, I'll be dead in a little over a year?"

The doctor didn't say a word but maintained her gaze looking directly into my eyes. A slow but deliberate nod of her head confirmed my interpretation. She went on presenting some other numbers, treatment options, and possibilities but I didn't hear those. The 1.1 number stuck and that was the object of my focus.

What great news!

I might have another entire year to live! Maybe more with treatment! If cancer were the cause of my death, it would give me more time than I was expecting.

Now tell me, in what frame of mind does a person have to be to interpret one year to live as good news?

I had to look up and over my right shoulder to see how Cindy was taking the news. She was devastated and couldn't stop the flow of tears. She studied me to see how I was reacting and wondered why I displayed a sense of calm and relief. I may have just discovered the mystery of how I would meet my demise. There was an outlook beyond "at any moment" for my time left on this earth. That was a step in a workable direction and provided a little more clarity.

Cindy was now receiving hugs and sympathy wishes from the tearful nurses in the hematology unit. The doctor had dismissed herself and left us to process the diagnosis with some printed information about MDS. Our homework assignment was to decide among three potential treatment options presented by the doctor. Neither Cindy nor I understood much of what she said the options were or what she recommended. We would have to try to make some sense of them later after we got our arms around the diagnosis.

We walked to the car in silence holding hands. How was I going to spin this? There was no way I could say everything was going to be alright. Or, "don't worry I've got this." Or, "we'll find a way to get through it." I choked back my typical go-to response of "we've been through worse than this." It didn't apply. There was no credible answer to her question, "what do we do now?"

What do you do immediately after a cancer diagnosis? Where do you go? What do you say? You go to Sweet Tomatoes for lunch, of course. Somehow, it seemed right to have our next conversations over lunch doing what we would typically do. And with dessert included, we could drown our sorrows with bowls of chocolate and vanilla ice cream swirls drenched in warm chocolate sauce.

I felt a strange sense of relief after the diagnosis and some difficult conversations with Cindy. The cat was out of the bag. I could talk about the limited number of my days with my best friend. The weight of keeping the secret of my pending demise was off my shoulders. All I had to do was tell her the rest of the story. Should I do that now? Or, had she been through enough already? She was reeling from the diagnosis. Maybe it's best to get it over with and deal with all the bad news at once. I was forming the thoughts in my mind, but I couldn't put them into words. I kicked the can down the road a little further to allow more time to get our arms around life as a cancer patient. I didn't add the weight of the revelation to the dreadful news we received that day. A better day would come, and I'd tell her then.

Our daughters knew of my condition and the doctor's appointment and were waiting to hear the results. We wanted some time to process the information but couldn't postpone the task of telling them about the diagnosis. I maintained my supernatural sense of calm and God-given peace throughout those difficult conversations which helped me get through them. Other than our two daughters, we kept the news to ourselves until we had a better handle on things and knew more about the treatment plan.

Decision time. On a journey such as this, there are many forks in the road. Many of the required decisions fall in the life or death category. They can mean extending the quality of life or bringing about premature death. Now, we had to make one of those decisions. Do we stick with the clinic that made the diagnosis and pursue treatment there or seek a second opinion? The clinic was nearby. The staff was well qualified. They did find the cancer after all. Did I want to go through all those painful tests again? Shouldn't they be the ones I lean on for treatment?

This decision came quickly. Cindy was adamant about getting a second opinion. The hematologist mentioned it in passing, and we decided to move on it. Besides, we had one of the best cancer hospitals in the world right in our backyard. The University of Texas MD Anderson Cancer Center sits in the heart of Houston's Medical Center, a collection of over 50 medical institutions in about three-square miles just south of downtown Houston. It's the largest medical complex in the world and one of the things Houston residents brag about. I'd be in good company as over 5,000,000 patients are treated in Medical Center facilities each year. After a few phone calls and an exchange of paperwork, I set the first appointment. It didn't take long. A guy with an MDS diagnosis was a high priority.

April 13, Day -427

The MD Anderson Cancer Center is a vast complex all by itself. There are over a dozen buildings many of which are connected by sky bridges and walkways. The first visit was a daunting experience and difficult to navigate, but we were able to find our way to the Leukemia Center on the 8th floor of the main building. Fortunately, the staff gives first-time visitors and rookies like us an extra touch of care and assistance getting to the right place at the right time. That first day was a blur of doctor visits and a flurry of tests that included, yes, another dreaded bone marrow biopsy.

There wasn't much time to ponder the circumstances or ask ourselves why we were here. It's like running from class to class in a new high school where everything is unfamiliar and getting from place to place takes twice as long as it should. The sight of thousands of other cancer patients waiting for tests, appointments or treatments had a profound impact. Yes, thousands. The parking garage was full. Elevators were crowded. People scurried everywhere. Many patients were sleeping in waiting room chairs. Many got from place to place in wheelchairs guided by friends or family members. Many patients displayed bald heads, a slight build, drooping shoulders and a discernable lack of energy. I could see their suffering, and I grieved for them.

I was feeling guilty and a little awkward standing upright and walking briskly with a full head of hair. While most patients bore visible scars of their cancer battles, I could be identified only by the official MDA wristband bearing my name, date of birth and medical number. In a sad attempt to show I was "one of them" I made sure my wristband was always visible. I felt a little better about smiling and greeting others as a patient who might understand rather than a visitor or caregiver who knew nothing of their struggles. I would learn more and more about those struggles as time went on and how my pity was not needed and grossly misplaced.

We had a few days to kill between the second round of testing and our appointment with the doctor to get the results. The hole in my hip halted the running schedule while I healed from the second bone marrow biopsy. I now had matching puncture wounds on both sides of my posterior. There was plenty to talk about with Cindy, however, and conversations while walking along the Waterway were never plagued with awkward silence. What if the first diagnosis was wrong? What if the new tests were unable to identify any cancer at all? Since I still had no symptoms of any illness, I held out that possibility. I will meet my maker soon anyway, but I didn't feel like a guy with bone marrow cancer. Cindy was hanging on to the hope that the initial diagnosis was a terrible mistake and that this was merely the beginning of a horrible dream.

April 20, Day -420

After successfully negotiating the MD Anderson labyrinth one more time we found ourselves sitting in a chilly examination room waiting for the doctor. Even though the wait could be quite a while, there was nothing to help you pass the time. No coffee, magazines or paperback books. Comfort was not a consideration in this room. It was all business. There were no personal items like pictures of family members, birthday cards or vacation mementos. Instructive signs describing what not to do took their place. Don't fall or don't leave without telling a nurse. Clean up crews were sure to erase any history in this room. No windows, no furniture, and no pictures hung on the faded lavender and beige walls that were meant to be soothing and peaceful. It didn't work. We were nervous with a long list of questions that had been building for weeks.

Cindy fidgeted, and I looked around the room for something I could adjust, play with or examine. If you were in this cave, you wanted to be somewhere else, and the idea of a quick escape was tempting. But we were here for a reason. We had a list of questions, and Dr. Steven Kornblau would be here any minute now and deliver the answers.

A Google search after our last visit unearthed an impressive resume. Kornblau was a Professor (with tenure) in the departments of Leukemia and Stem Cell Transplantation. Dr. Kornblau did his hematology and oncology fellowship training at MDA and had been on staff since 1991. He has received international recognition for his research in Acute Myeloid Leukemia cell biology. God placed me in his patient's chair, right where I was supposed to be. Dr. Kornblau knew his stuff and would either confirm the previous diagnosis or tell us it had all been an unfortunate misunderstanding.

A casual knock on the exam room door announced his entrance followed by two nurses who found it difficult to find some breathing room in such a small space. Dr. Kornblau wasn't just the smartest person in the room; he probably ran circles around everyone in the building. I could see him at the podium announcing research results at a fancy doctors' conference. He could easily command the attention of other doctors and hold their interest while laying out a stack of tedious details. He was more than capable of multitasking, and he might have been thinking about his next presentation, but his attention was directly on me. Out of thousands of patients crowding the waiting rooms at MD Anderson, his focus gave me the impression that my case was important. I was important. We locked eyes, and I didn't resist his probing looks at both Cindy and me seemingly to determine how best to deliver the news. His review of all those tests and the ream of data that they produced were about to be announced. I braced myself for the big reveal hoping for some good news.

No such luck. The results were conclusive. It was Myelodysplastic Syndrome. I had bone marrow cancer. Dr. Kornblau's gentle but firm summary of the test results left no doubt. After confirming the diagnosis, he went directly into the treatment plan. Kornblau didn't present a list of options to consider or decisions to contemplate. He made only one recommendation which I greatly appreciated. His white lab coat and graying temples reinforced his status as the captain of this ship, and we were happy he was at the helm. Chemotherapy was recommended to kill off some of the cancerous stem cells, bring the blast countdown to a level well below 20%, and keep me from progressing into AML. He clearly stated that his plan was not a cure. His program was intended to slow the progression of the disease and improve the quality of life I had remaining. Perhaps it would extend my life for a few more years. I was certainly up for that.

Beyond that, there was only one way to eradicate or "cure" the disease. A Stem Cell Transplant might kill the subpar bone marrow in my body along with the cancerous stem cells and replace them with new ones from a healthy donor. It's a risky "Hail Mary" procedure but one we may want to consider depending on the success or failure of the chemotherapy treatments. The other transplant details eluded us as we contemplated the treatments at hand.

Dr. Kornblau's recommended plan included monthly chemotherapy treatment cycles of 7 days. I would receive a treatment each day for seven consecutive days. After a three-week break, the next seven-day cycle would begin.

"How long will we have to do this?" Cindy asked hoping for a short term.

One of the nurses fielded this question, and the answer hit both of us like a punch we didn't see coming.

"Forever," was the matter of fact reply. "If we stop the treatments, the cancerous stem cells would return to the previous level or progress further."

The cycles would repeat monthly for the rest of my life. We had taken some punches, but this one landed with full force deep in the gut. I didn't ask any more questions for fear of more answers like that.

Both Dr. Kornblau and his assistant assured us that the prescribed chemotherapy drug was not extremely harsh and that many patients tolerated it without much disruption to their lives. That didn't make the life sentence any easier to accept. Another upbeat and well-qualified nurse suggested that we consider these cycles our "new normal." That is such a horrible phrase. The new normal. Both Cindy and I learned to despise that term. For us, it never meant anything good. It signaled a painful adaptation to another lousy set of circumstances.

While the doctor and nurses were reluctant to make a prognosis, I had to know and kept pushing for an answer.

"What is my life expectancy if I follow this plan?" I pressed. "How long do I have?"

Finally, Dr. Kornblau looked me in the eye and gave me the prognosis.

"Three to five years."

What? Three to five years? That was great news! The date of my demise had gone from "soon" to 1.1 years to three to five years. I liked this prognosis much better than the initial one. Cindy is having trouble coping with another agonizing punch in the gut. I was excited about the additional year or two to live. God may have other plans, but it seemed like a natural conclusion that the course of this disease fit into the definition of "soon." And, again, what kind of perspective does one have to have to receive a prognosis of three to five years and consider it good news?

Spending the rest of my life as a cancer patient undergoing continuous chemotherapy treatments didn't sound like much fun even with a relatively mild chemo drug. Agreeing to the treatment plan was not automatic. If I was being called home soon anyway, why go through the treatments at all? Why not take my chances and let the MDS take its course? Maybe it won't progress into Acute Myeloid Leukemia. Maybe God is directing me to face squarely any new symptoms or complications. Maybe I should just be happy with the knowledge of how I would meet my demise. Dr. Kornblau made the appointment for the first chemotherapy treatment, but I wasn't 100% sure that was the way I would go. A decision like this required some contemplation and a lot of prayer.

What would you do?

Conventional wisdom would take you down the medical path and begin the treatment plan immediately preventing a turn for the worse. Spiritual wisdom might suggest placing yourself in God's hands and letting Him handle any complications that may arise. A cowardly decision might be sidestepping the treatment plan altogether, avoiding the pain and discomfort and accepting whatever fate may bring.

It wasn't as clear as a lightning bolt, a burning bush or another revelation but God led me in the direction of conventional medical wisdom. I didn't feel a compulsion to reject the doctors' recommendations and take a stand. I had no fear of the treatments. When I asked the question in prayer, I received a calming sense. Take the treatments. Do it with a positive outlook. Let God's light and hope shine brightly in a place where it is so desperately needed. Be an inspiration to others. Provide a friendly face. Let God work through my weakness. Learn to depend entirely on God's strength, patience, and peace.

Would you do that? Could you do that? Could you place your life and health entirely in God's hands?

I'm glad I didn't know how bumpy or wild it would be. But I buckled my proverbial seat belt and went along for the ride.

The new treatment plan and a new life as a cancer patient would begin in one week.

Chapter 4

Acceptance

I'm now on borrowed time. It's been eight months since the revelation and God did His part. He gave me a few months to work out the issues we had negotiated. God more than fulfilled the terms or spirit of that agreement. He hasn't hinted at any extensions. He hasn't given me any indication that there will be any additional years, months or even days to live. It's one day at a time at this point.

It has taken all of these eight months to get my arms around these circumstances and to understand where I am and accept it. I'm going home soon. I have bone marrow cancer. If that's where I am, that's where I am. I accept it. I own it. I am thankful for it. Wait a minute. Thankful? Seriously? As crazy as that sounds, yes. I am thankful. Seriously. God has a plan for my life and will somehow use this disease for His good purpose and my greater good. He is transforming my thought process and expanding my heart to more deeply feel the plight of others. He is preparing me for something, but at this point, I don't know what it is.

That kind of acceptance and thanksgiving isn't anything I would naturally come by on my own. That kind of acceptance and the peace that comes with it comes from God. The Holy Spirit provides the supernatural ability to accept these circumstances and praise God in all things and at all times. I am thankful for it, cling to it and wrap myself in it. That acceptance sets me free. I don't have to fight the diagnosis. I don't have to harbor any denial. I don't have to complain that it happened to me or even wonder why. It just did.

Now, I can deal with it. Now, I can look forward, not backward. Now I can wonder, what's next?

Acceptance makes it much easier to talk openly with family and friends. And, now that the doctors had confirmed the diagnosis and outlined a treatment plan, it was time to share that information with others. The acceptance and peace I had with the diagnosis and the road ahead would make it much easier to describe the type of cancer I was to battle, what that battle may look like and how I was going to fight it. It will make it easier for other people to communicate openly and feel free to ask the questions they may want to ask. If I'm comfortable talking about the subject, they may be more comfortable with it, too.

Whether I wanted to tell them or not, I was forced to communicate directly with my siblings. During all the preparation for the chemotherapy treatments, I also was being prepared for the possibility of a Stem Cell Transplant which is a long lead time item. The search would have to begin now as locating a suitable donor with an exact tissue match would take some time. Ultimately, the best chance for a donor match is a brother or a sister.

I put off reaching out to my sister and three brothers, but a doctor at MD Anderson charged with the task of finding related donors kept on me. He didn't accept my procrastination and saw through my delay tactics. Openly speaking of problems or issues I faced was not my forte. Usually, I would bring up a topic like this after the treatments were well underway and I could talk about some results. I didn't want to have this conversation now. Not this early in the treatment process. First, I had to tell my siblings about the diagnosis and then ask them for their blood. Literally. How could I do that? At the time, that concept was inconceivable.

I needed a strategy, or so I thought so I hatched a diabolical plot was where I would pass along the bad news and wait for them to ask if there was anything they could do. People always say that.

42

Then, bam! I would say that there WAS something they could do. Submit to a blood test and send the sample to MD Anderson. Cindy challenged that conclusion and pointed out that I had no need for a strategy or plot. I should take a simple step. Let them know what was going on and ask for their help. Easy for her to say. I would give myself a barely passing grade on helping others and a failing grade at asking people for help. Even a close relative. But, of course, she was right. And, as time would progress, I would learn how to empathize more with the challenges of others and accept the help I needed.

My weapon of choice was email. Since none of my immediate family lived in the Houston area, a face to face conversation was off the table. Writing would allow me to cover the necessary details of Myelodysplastic Syndrome and how it interferes with the production of white blood cells. And, it would give me the chance to explain the need for a blood sample and what the stem cell donation process would entail. An email would allow me to get everything on the table and prevent leaving out some key details. All four siblings would get the same complete story. I had to refer to my stack of pamphlets and worksheets provided by M D Anderson to fill the gaps in my knowledge to accurately cover everything that needed to be said. The research process helped complete my education and would help me explain when the inevitable follow up telephone calls were made.

April 25, Day -415

Here is the text of the email sent to my older brother Mike:

Mike,

I know I should have said something over the weekend in our telephone conversation or text messages. But I didn't want to put a damper on your family party or be a distraction on your birthday.

But I have some news and a request. Neither of which is pleasant. But, instead of a phone call out of left field, I thought it best to give you an overview in email form first.

I have cancer.

I got a red flag in March with an advanced stage of Myelodysplastic Syndrome (MDS), a rare form of bone marrow cancer. Bone marrow normally produces stem cells that turn into red blood cells, white blood cells, and platelets that move into the bloodstream. My bone marrow is out of whack and the stem cells aren't maturing into healthy blood cells.

I got that red flag during a routine physical last October. My blood test showed extremely low levels of white blood cells. Follow up monthly blood tests showed a decline in red blood cells and platelets. The MDS diagnosis was made after a bone marrow biopsy last month. Fortunately, the world-renowned MD Anderson Cancer Center is right down the road here in Houston. After another round of tests, they confirmed the MDS diagnosis. They developed a treatment plan that includes chemotherapy and a clinical trial of a drug that may improve the success rate.

The goal is to kill off the immature stem cells that are hampering the normal production of healthy blood cells. If they can get them low enough then I should be able to manage the cancer. The treatments start this week, and they should know in four to six months if the chemotherapy is working. It's a 50/50 shot but my age (young for this type of cancer) and good health work to my advantage.

If all else fails, a stem cell transplant may be necessary. That's where they take out all my crappy stem cells and replace them with normal ones.

And, thus, the request. The best normal stem cells come from siblings. My doctor has requested that I check with you and the other siblings to see if there is a match determined by a simple blood test. It takes a lot of time to locate non-related donors, so they are pushing me to start knocking on doors now.

A stem cell transplant is the last thing I want to have. For me, it's a high-risk procedure with no guarantee of success. It requires many days in the hospital and a long recovery period. For the donor, it's ten days in Houston. They get shots for a couple of days to stimulate stem cell production and push the stem cells out of the bone marrow and into the bloodstream. The stem cells are filtered from the blood over a several day period in a process called apheresis. The blood goes out through an IV, into a machine where the stem cells are collected, then the rest of the blood goes back to the donor. The side effects are minimal, but the injections can be painful, and the IV's don't sound like much fun.

If you are willing to take this on, let me know. I'll pass your contact information along to MD Anderson. They will follow up with details on the blood test and more information on the donor process. MD Anderson covers all the costs involved.

Again, a stem cell transplant is the last resort. It would only be considered if the chemotherapy doesn't work and the cancer gets worse.

Marc
(I was never one for flashy salutations.)

A flood of nerves overloaded my system as soon as I hit the "send" button on the computer screen. I hadn't discussed cancer with anyone but Cindy, my daughters, and the medical professionals. The email I just sent would begin the process of telling who knows how many people about a rare and unfamiliar cancer. Only about 12,500 cases of Myelodysplastic Syndrome are diagnosed each year compared to 200,000 annual cases diagnosed for more common cancers like lung or breast cancer. I would have to explain the normal process of stem cell production in the bone marrow, how those cells mature into healthy red and white blood cells and how MDS screws up that process. By attacking the mutant stem cells, the chemotherapy treatments are expected to lower the percentage of mutant cells allowing more of the healthy ones to mature and move into the bloodstream. However, I knew my stuff. I had the facts. I did the homework. I'm ready for the conversations. A piece of cake, right?

Before that flood of nerves had settled, the cell phone sitting on the coffee table lit up. Brother Mike was on the phone. He would be my first test. Could I hold it together? Could I adequately explain what was going on? Could I keep him from worrying? Mike wasn't an email or text message kind of guy. Nor was he the kind of guy to procrastinate or think things completely through. He would typically face tough issues head-on, right now and preferably face to face. He was the older brother and the first male child of our family, after all.

"Hey, big boy. What the heck?" were the first words from Mike and the first from my family. The language was cleaned up a bit for more sensitive readers.

The conversation was the first of its kind. The McCoy family had some bouts with various illnesses but nothing terminal. Other than my father who struggled with heart disease most of his adult life, my immediate family members had good genes and managed to stay out of hospitals. All were living, breathing and healthy. I was the first to contract something serious and life-threatening.

The call went better than I thought it would. Some deep gulps held back the flood of nerves and emotions lying just below the surface. The peace I held so tightly was in ample supply and kept me on task. I knew the diagnosis well and was able to relay it factually. Mike remained in older brother mode listening carefully, asking good questions and offering more than enough comforting advice even though I can't remember what it was. I can only remember the feeling of support and encouragement. He expressed immediately his "all in" status as a potential donor available any place at any time. As I reflect on that conversation, what remains is how much he cared and his willingness to go out of his way, way out of his way, to help me any way he could. I felt loved. I felt like he cared. Lots of words flew back and forth, but it's that feeling that lives in my memory.

Conversations with other family members went the same way. There were some awkward moments where they didn't know what to say, and I didn't always get facts straight, but the result was usually the same. Their love, concern, and compassion came through loud and clear. And that was the best medicine. Those feelings were always there over the years but not always stated and not always received. The cancer diagnosis brought them to the forefront. And that's one of the benefits of going through a crisis like this. Conversations become much more meaningful and feelings that might usually be withheld jump right to center stage.

What I was learning would be strongly reinforced over the next few months. Those things that used to be important were quickly fading away while relationships shone brightly. Getting a good deal on a car or having the latest version of the iPhone doesn't have much meaning when you're not going to be around long. Relationships, however, grow in value, retain the most meaning and become the top priority.

What if there is no tomorrow? What would take on more importance in your life or become meaningless? What would you choose to do today?

Usually, we don't think like that. We have time. Plenty of time. That project can wait until tomorrow. I'll be a better person tomorrow. I'll read more scripture and get started tomorrow. I'll get in shape someday. Maybe tomorrow. I'll spend more time with the kids once I complete this big project at work. Not tomorrow but someday soon, wink, wink.

If there is no tomorrow, no someday, what would retain priority status in your life?

As each day dawned, the answer to that question became more and more clear. Material things weren't important at all. Those desires fell away quickly. There was nothing unfinished or unresolved in my former career and certainly nothing significant enough to devote any time to now. The applause and attention I enjoyed in previous years from doing something exceptional or finishing first lost their appeal. I would typically enjoy being the center of attention, but even that inclination was fading quickly. It just didn't matter anymore.

Anything even remotely sinful was out of the question since I was meeting my maker soon. I couldn't justify or rationalize anything intentionally sinful in myself or that which might encourage another to sin. An intense desire to deepen my knowledge of God, understand His purpose for these last few days and be obedient to God's will had taken its place. Good Christians always think of those things but from a different perspective. They can do them with the focus and intensity they deserve tomorrow. I didn't have that kind of time.

What grew, what bloomed, what changed was the way I interacted with other people. The critical thing that rose to number one on my priority list was those relationships. If there is no tomorrow what do you say to people today? How do you conduct yourself around people you don't know? How do you interact with people you love? There was surely no point in being rude or pushy. There was no point in leaving a negative impression with anyone. Why frown when you can smile? Why be shy when you can introduce yourself and say something encouraging? Are you in a hurry or something? What are you waiting for? Tomorrow?

Why seek justice with your existing relationships? Why hold grudges? Why not relegate those things to the past and focus on the way the relationship should be today? Again, what are you waiting for? Tomorrow?

Why not enjoy the love, common interests and shared experiences you have with friends and family? Most likely, they will respond to your actions. They may scratch their heads and wonder what you're up to, but they are apt to play along. Why not give it a shot? What's the worst that could happen? And, why wait for a later time?

The most precious relationship I have on this earth is with Cindy. I fell hopelessly in love the moment I saw her over 40 years ago. The love has survived and prospered for decades and continues to develop. Even though I didn't think our love could get any stronger or deeper, I felt it taking on yet another dimension. I wasn't shaping it. It was shaping me. The love I felt for Cindy shifted into a new gear, and all I wanted to do was spend time with her. I had no bucket list. No experiences I needed to have, goals to reach or conquests to make. I just wanted to spend the time I had with her. If I had a week, a month or a few short minutes, I wanted them to be in her presence.

As I moved through this journey and savored each of my remaining days, all my relationships changed for the better and much more love came to the forefront. Distant acquaintances came closer. I heard from friends more often. Strained relationships became more relaxed. Strong relationships became even stronger. New relationships were welcome and cherished. People expressed their love for me, and I wasn't afraid or hesitant to say that I loved them. Love took on a more active role. More than a feeling, it was a matter of doing things to express that love. It's amazing how the way you look at people changes and how others look at you changes when time is short, and there is no tomorrow. Wouldn't it be great if everyone lived every moment as if there were no tomorrow?

My life had been turned inside out and upside down. I didn't look at anything the same as I did a few short months ago. Each sunrise was more striking. Birds in flight appeared more graceful. The muddy waterway seemed cleaner. Bumper to bumper traffic was less annoying. Cindy looked hotter. Keep in mind that none of those things or people had changed. The way I looked at them had changed, and I came to appreciate the difference.

It took a large-scale revelation and a cancer diagnosis to bring about this new perspective, but it was one of the benefits of living a life compressed into a year or two. It was one of the benefits of giving up the struggle with my circumstances. Once I had accepted my diagnosis and my new lifestyle, I was free to move past them and fully embrace and appreciate the benefits.

And, as if I needed more change in my life, I was about to embark on a physical makeover. The revelation changed my attitude. Chemotherapy was about to change my body.

Chapter 5
Chemotherapy

April 27, Day -413

Chemo weeks are tough. They require seven applications of a drug called Azacitidine commonly referred to by its brand name Vidaza. The drug is applied intravenously once per day for seven consecutive days. Each IV infusion takes roughly two hours and requires a trip to the Ambulatory Treatment Center at MD Anderson.

Azacitidine, or Vidaza, targets the cancerous stem cells produced by bone marrow and inhibits their growth. As you can imagine it wreaks havoc in many other areas as well resulting in side effects such as nausea, vomiting, dizziness, fatigue, fevers and both diarrhea and constipation. Figure that one out.

Whenever I would ask a doctor, nurse or any other medical professional what side effects I will experience, the answer is always the same.

"It depends," they would say. I heard a variation of that reply every time I asked the question. "Everyone is different and experiences therapies differently."

In other words, they don't know. They can give you statistics, averages, and descriptions of others' experiences but they can't tell you how you will react. I must have heard that a thousand times. At first, I thought they were dodging the question. I came to learn,

53

however, that it was true. They don't know. Each body reacts differently. The unpredictability is frustrating, but it's just the way it is.

How would I react to 150 mg of Azacitidine injected directly into my vein? It depends. It's never been done. Not to me, anyway. We'll have to wait and see. I did receive one warning from a medical professional. They told me not to drive after the infusion.

With that assurance, Cindy accompanied me to my first chemotherapy treatment at MD Anderson. After checking in at the desk and getting a wristband identifying me by name, birthdate and medical record number, we strolled into the large open waiting area to listen for a nurse to call my name. The waiting area could accommodate about 100 people and was near capacity most of the time. It felt more like a busy library than a waiting room. It was a quiet place void of the noisy conversations you expect to hear from a large group of people. The unspoken and unwritten rule was to keep it down and show some respect for those around you.

Among the patients in the ATC, I felt guilty again. They were feeling horrible, and I was feeling fine. I still didn't have any symptoms associated with my MDS and other than being a bundle of nerves, I felt healthy and strong. I still felt the need to let people know I was a patient, so I made sure my wristband was clearly visible. I didn't want people to think I was a visitor with all this energy and little respect for the plight of others struggling with their treatments.

A look around the waiting area at the Ambulatory Treatment Center can break your heart. Many patients are laying on couches covered with blankets resting after their treatments. Many others are in obvious pain seated in recliners unable to leave until the side effects subside. Most look weak and exhausted. Patients like me waiting for treatments didn't exhibit much happiness, either. Most seemed weary dreading the discomfort they were soon to face.

These patients didn't have many options. The only reason they would endure the mutilation and poisoning of their bodies is that the alternative is even more frightful. They may be a shell of what they used to be, but they are still alive and fighting for every breath. The pity I felt during my first visit was fading fast. Deep respect was growing as I came to see my fellow patients as fighters, warriors and a special breed of courageous people. I hope I have a fraction of their superhuman strength. I hope I can summon the kind of courage they have when it comes time for me to face the physical tests that lie ahead.

Pack a lunch or bring a good book to keep you occupied while you wait. It could be as little as 30 minutes or as long as a couple of hours before you are called back for your treatment. Cheerful volunteers with comforting smiles, many of whom were cancer survivors themselves, would stop by and say hello offering coffee, tea, crackers or cookies. If you asked them a question or initiated a conversation, they would drop everything and happily oblige. Otherwise, they would allow you to maintain your space and keep working to empty their carts. Individually wrapped peppermints were always a big hit as they tended to settle the stomach and take the inevitable and nasty medicine taste out of a patient's mouth.

Like a good sports bar, there are plenty of TV screens around but watching the replay of a golf match, or a daytime television talk show didn't have much appeal. We were nervously surveying the room looking for clues to what we were about to experience. We found a couple of loungers far from the TV screens. They faced a floor to ceiling window overlooking the front entrance of the Cancer Center. The natural light would make it easier to read, but we were too nervous to try. We let the time pass watching people coming and going at the main entrance. One observation became crystal clear. A lot of people are struggling with cancer of one type or another. Some walk in the door. Others ride in wheelchairs. Most have the telltale sign of a bald head. I rubbed my full head of hair wondering how long it would survive the chemotherapy.

Patients come to MD Anderson from all over the world, speak many different languages, and display all types of dress. While we all look so different, we have one thing in common. We have a catastrophic illness, and we're hoping to eke out a few more years or be one of the select few that survive and maybe even fully recover. Our body language communicates the pain and anguish of the treatments, and the hope and optimism revealed in raised eyebrows or a simple smile. Our shared experience binds us and overrides all the other experiences that separate us.

"McCoy!"

The nurse stepped out of the infusion area and interrupted my thoughts of unity and world peace. You could hear that call from the next county. My time was at hand.

"McCoy!"

We rose quickly and hurried over to the door to acknowledge that I was, in fact, McCoy. Not knowing the protocol, we didn't want to risk losing our place if we didn't get there quickly enough.

"Medical record number?"

I hadn't memorized it yet and had to check my wristband. Once I proved my identity the nurse led me to the vital signs station to make sure I could handle the treatment. No fever. Oxygen levels in my blood were excellent. My elevated heart rate and blood pressure didn't alarm anyone. They must expect that from a nervous rookie.

"Follow me to room 38. Do you want a warm blanket?"

Do I need one, I wondered?

"That sounds great, thank you," I said trying to convey my appreciation without sounding like a rookie. I decided to go with the blanket offer since it was chilly, and I wanted to prepare for anything. Here's some good advice. Never turn down a warm blanket.

Room 38 was a typical small clinic room with a twin sized bed and a side chair under a white and sterile overhead light. The lavender and yellow beige walls looked familiar. I took a chair as I observed the collection of medical equipment crowding the space locking on the "tree" beside the bed. Plastic bags with drugs in liquid form would soon hang on that tall rolling stand with the force of gravity directing their flow into my arm. When more precision was needed a mechanical pump the size of a big shoebox bolted to the trunk would regulate the dosage and rate of flow. I would get well acquainted with the mechanics of this "tree" over the next few months.

The nurse dressed in scrubs came in shortly after our arrival. She knew it was our first IV treatment and went out of her way to make us feel comfortable. Her confidence was reassuring. Fortunately, it wasn't her first rodeo. In Texas, that bit of slang is high praise and a strong compliment.

I climbed into the hospital bed and adjusted the back to shape it more like a large recliner than a bed. It seemed like it was barely above freezing in the room and I'm glad I had the warm blankets to cover my body and shoulders. My arm had to be free and available for the IV needle, so it stuck out from under the covers. It would just have to be cold.

The nurse tied a piece of elastic around the bicep closest to the IV tree and tapped some veins in my arm trying to coax one to the surface. Before I knew it, she skillfully inserted the needle on the inside of my left forearm and taped it down. It pinched a little, but the pain didn't last long. The nurse connected that needle to a thin plastic hose with lots of valves on it that ran up to the top of the tree where the hooks held the bags of liquid. A bag of saline the size of a thick paperback book had the task of keeping the line open while the pharmacist prepared the chemo drugs. The cooling sensation of the liquid entering the vein woke me up but faded after a few minutes. The nurse returned with the second bag of liquid called Zofran administered about 30 minutes before the Azacitidine to minimize nausea. That's good stuff and keeps you from throwing up after the chemo treatment.

Azacitidine has a short shelf life. Only about 60 minutes. It has to be special ordered and prepared immediately before being administered. The nurse comes back in with the bag of recently mixed Azacitidine from the pharmacy followed by another nurse to verify the drug, the order, the dosage, and the patient. Both nurses are now wearing chemo gowns resembling hazmat suits over their scrubs to prevent any accidental contact with the Azacitidine. It's hazardous for them to touch it but I guess it's okay to infuse it directly into my bloodstream. I took little comfort in that observation.

It's an easy connection to the infusion tubes, and the nurses are off to tend to another patient. Cindy and I are looking at each other while the bags are dripping, and the pump is pumping. The treatment is underway, and there is no turning back now. How would I react? It depends. Who knows? No one knows. We'll have to wait and see.

Little by little the bags of fluid get smaller and smaller. It's an exact two-hour infusion, and I don't think I moved a muscle the entire time. The exposed arm, hand and fingers were freezing, but I was afraid to move them. I didn't want to pull on the needle in any way. Anytime a person got even close to the plastic tube I was afraid they would trip and yank it out of my arm. Cindy and I had a nervous conversation for the better part of those two hours sharing thoughts about this strange experience and how we ultimately found ourselves in this position.

Once the last drop of fluid made its way through the plastic tube and entered my arm, the nurse removed the needle. I rubbed my near frozen limb and tried to get some extra blood flowing to my icy fingers. Then, I gave myself a mental pat down trying to determine how the chemo drugs had affected me. I was groggy and lightheaded, but I wasn't sure if it was due to the infusion or laying down for three hours in the middle of the day. I struggled as I stood up, donned my jacket, took Cindy's outstretched hand and headed for the exit. That was after the nurse reminded me again not to try to drive home.

That was the first of 91 such treatments I would endure over the next 13 months. The process got much easier with experience. I learned how to work the TV, adjust the bed and control the lighting in the rooms. I discovered I could move my arm around and the little sliver of plastic under my skin wouldn't go anywhere. I learned not to eat or drink anything before the infusions, so I wouldn't have to go to the bathroom in the middle of the process. Several infusion centers served patients throughout the MD Anderson complex, and we got to know each one of them. After watching other patients rolling their trees down the hall, I learned that you could unplug the pump and shift it to battery power. Freedom! I could roll the tree up and down the hallways to stretch my legs and steer it to the bathroom if I had to go. That's life changing information, folks.

Cindy and I got to know some of the other patients with similar IV treatment schedules and were even able to help some of the newer patients get more familiar with the process. The massive MD Anderson complex was getting smaller and smaller as we got to know our way around. After a while, we could tell you how to locate the best little restaurants, how to find the strongest cup of coffee and how to take advantage of the schedule flexibility if we needed to move some appointments around.

The side effects of each treatment were not pleasant. Nausea hit me hard and the fatigue even harder. My body was weak, and I struggled to hold the contents of my stomach. The sight of food made me feel even sicker. There wasn't much I could do after the treatments but lay on the couch and try to sleep it off. The first two or three days of each cycle weren't so bad but the last two days and the two days following the cycles were much more difficult. The side effects got worse as each day of the cycle progressed, and by the seventh day, it felt like getting hit with a cruel hangover and a severe case of the flu at the same time.

We learned quickly not to schedule anything we could avoid during chemo week. I didn't have the strength or the will to go many places or do much of anything. Church activities were different. I'd do whatever I had to do to attend a men's group meeting, an afternoon Bible study or a Sunday morning service. After the two-day recovery period, we'd try to get back to "normal" and enjoy the three weeks between treatment cycles. That's when we could meet up with friends, attend a live music event or entertain visitors. And, just when I'd start to feel like I was getting close to 80 to 90% of my normal self, it was time for the next cycle.

Here we go again. Time to adapt. I had to accept that this was my "new normal" (we detest that term) and that this was how I was to live for the remaining weeks, months or years God would give me. There is no cure for MDS, and there was no end to the chemotherapy treatments. If you want three to five extra years, this is the price you had to pay. Weighing all the alternatives and receiving the inspiration from those fellow fighters in the MD Anderson waiting rooms, I chose to adapt and deal with it.

As a few months passed, I realized how much physical change there would be and how much adaptation would have to take place.

Chemotherapy changes everything physically. Mentally, you feel the same. But, from the neck down it feels like someone replaced your body. The new body is similar to the old body, but it doesn't work quite the same. The saliva tastes different. You sneeze differently. Your skin feels different to the touch. Bathroom functions are no longer the same. Even breathing feels awkward and the air moving in and out of your lungs has a different texture to it. There is no doubt it is your body. It's just different, and it takes some effort to adjust to the changes.

Then there were "The Tingles," the most lasting of my new physical attributes. When I perspire, it feels like hundreds of tiny pinpricks poke the skin from the inside out. They came without warning. Nobody wrote about The Tingles in any pamphlet or brochure. No doctors or nurses mentioned that side effect. The first time I felt The Tingles I was trying to get some exercise between chemotherapy treatments. My skin wanted to let some perspiration loose, but it seemed like my pores were stuck. The perspiration seemed to be thicker than it used to be and clogged up those pores. Only a good sweat would generate enough pressure to push the clogs through the pores. Imagine getting a golf ball stuck in a garden hose. If you have kids, you know it could happen. Turn up the water pressure high enough, and you might be able to push it through. The Tingles feel like that moment when golf balls shoot out of the end of a thousand hoses at the same time. Every time I sweat, I can count on a case of The Tingles.

I continued to exercise every day in spite of The Tingles alternating days between running and lifting weights. I had to slow down the pace of my runs and reduce the weights I would lift, but I kept going. I could hear my doctor's voice saying my job was to keep myself in as good physical condition as possible. He said I was the only cancer patient he had that could run six miles and as challenging as it was to motivate myself, I didn't want to give up that status.

I'd try to exercise on the first few days of each chemo cycle, but that didn't always work out. I had gotten used to The Tingles and could usually fight through nausea, but the dizziness was severe, and there would be many times I felt like I would pass out. Typically, I'd take chemo week off, rest for a day or two after the cycle then get back out for a slow run. I'd try to do more each day building from that point. Starting and stopping an exercise routine each month had its challenges, but I felt compelled to do whatever I could. I may not be running any half marathons soon, but I could at least maintain some level of physical conditioning. I knew deep down that the strength I got from exercise helped me fight through the side effects of chemotherapy.

And, there is nothing like a good 50-minute run. It clears your head, stretches your muscles, works your lungs, and you can count on The Tingles to flush your skin. It also provides some time for yourself to enjoy the natural surroundings and think things through. I'd recall incidents in my past like mistakes I'd made or choices I'd like to take back that resulted in uncomfortable circumstances or things I wish I wouldn't have said. Those regrettable events seemed critical at the time but felt so distant and unimportant now. I found it healthy and therapeutic to let those things go.

I talked to God frequently during those runs. I'd meditate on scripture I had read recently, or a sermon preached at church. Or, listen for instruction or allow space for new thoughts or ideas. While I wasn't necessarily searching for my purpose in this last phase of my life, I wanted to know and obey God's will. What I wanted wasn't important anymore. What good would that do? God's will was the top priority. I wanted to know His will for me today. Right now. Not tomorrow or in the long run. But right here and right now.

And, I wanted to be open to the conviction of the Holy Spirit. I frequently prayed that if there was anything in my life holding me back from obeying God's will or fully submitting myself to Him to bring it to my attention, so I could address it, change that behavior and seek His forgiveness. I learned to pay close attention to that feeling of uneasiness with a decision or the hair standing up on the back of my neck. It could be the Holy Spirit nudging me in a different direction. I could be sure I was proceeding in the right direction if I listened carefully, opened myself to God's will and didn't feel a conviction along the way.

I would ask God if there was a fast track to Christian maturity. After all, I had squandered many of my adult years striving for career and financial success thinking I'd get my spiritual act together "someday." I had been working on that for the past few years but still harbored a lot of remorse and wanted to make up for lost time. Someday was no longer an option. It was now or never. Did the revelation force me onto a faster track? I was learning, growing, changing, and evolving in a way that would have never been possible otherwise.

I felt sure in my purpose. I was a child of the Most High God here to serve and glorify Him. My job was to mature as a Christian seeking to be as much like Jesus as I could be before I passed away and became complete. The Holy Spirit led me to a scripture outlining what that process entailed.

In 2 Peter 1:3-4 we are called to godliness and to lean on God's promises to keep us from the corruption in the world.

"For this very reason, make every effort to add to your faith goodness; and to goodness, knowledge; and to knowledge, self-control; and to self-control, perseverance; and to perseverance, godliness; and to godliness, brotherly kindness; and to brotherly kindness, love." 2 Peter 1:5-7

That's a tall order and enough to keep a person busy for a long time. Love was a tough one and was at the pinnacle of that list. But love is the very essence of God and the basis for a mature Christian. That scripture became my focus and my "to-do" list for my remaining days.

I was also sure of my destination. My time on Earth was short, and I'd be moving on to eternal life soon. Jesus promised it. God created us for it. Eternal life was the ultimate reward to everyone who believed in God's Son and made Him their Lord and savior. And now, Heaven wasn't just a concept or something far far away. It was on my calendar and coming soon. I could be making a move from this world to that world any day at any time.

I should be ready to go but how do you prepare for a trip like that? I had a lot of questions but where do you find the answers? Was Heaven a real place? How would it look? How would I look? What would I do there? I had to know, and it was time I did some homework to find out.

Chapter 6

Heaven

"Coming face to face with my mortality
has awakened my appetite for eternity."
---Russ Ramsey from "So That I Might See"
The power of affliction in the Christian life.

Life is short. We hear that all the time, but we usually don't believe it. We think there is always tomorrow. We procrastinate. We wait for the timing to be right. We put things off especially the thought of our death. And, let's face it, we're afraid to die.

The mere thought of my passing was terrifying, and I tried to avoid it whenever I could. I'd even try to avoid funerals if I could come up with a good excuse. I sat through the funerals I felt obligated to attend and would tear up with all kinds of emotions even if I didn't know much about the person being eulogized. Funerals brought me face to face with my mortality and the inescapable vision of a funeral of my own. I could see my wife, my kids and my grandkids dressed in black sitting on the front row of the church. That scene was good for awkward tears every time. The image of a grandchild peeking over the edge of my casket to get one final look at Papa took me over the top.

With each passing year, the fear of death diminishes a little. Once you hit the golden age of 50 or 55, you start thinking about death from a different perspective. There are more days behind you than there are ahead of you. The end of our days becomes closer and closer as every day passes. Still, we tend to prepare for a long retirement rather than the short amount of time we have remaining.

The revelation and the cancer diagnosis put life and death in a new light. My perspective changed radically. Death wasn't something far off or something to deal with someday. It was imminent. It was soon. It was a certainty within three to five years. As Bob Dylan mumbled, I was "Knockin' on Heaven's Door."

As I read through the scriptures, any chapter or verse dealing with death jumped off the page. And there are plenty of them. As I took those scriptures to heart and embraced the concept of death, my interest in Heaven grew exponentially. I wanted the details. I wanted to know all about where I was going. The future wasn't full of possibilities or potential. The future was certain. I would meet my Savior in Heaven where I would reside until the end of days and our collective move to the New Jerusalem. That's going to happen soon.

But how does that eternity look? What will I do when I get there? What will I see? I had a deep desire to get some answers.

God wants us to know, too. Eternal life is the great promise of the Christian faith. It's our reward. It's our crown. It's our hope. He revealed much of Heaven to us in the book of Revelation through the apostle John. John was told to write down what was revealed to him "for these words are trustworthy and true."

If you want to know more about Heaven and your life eternal, go directly to the source that is trustworthy and true. The Bible clearly describes our new home in the New Jerusalem and the promise of our eternal life. Other commentaries and summaries can be helpful, but there is no substitute for the direct and unfiltered Word of God. Don't be afraid that you won't understand the flowery language or won't relate to a 2,000-year-old society. It's as relevant today as it was the day it was written. The Holy Spirit will guide you through it and provide the proper interpretation.

The Holy Spirit helped me convert the fuzzy concept of death to a vivid picture with me in it. As I read scripture with my short-term perspective, it became clear that Heaven was a real place and that we are citizens of Heaven and not of this earth. If we believe and overcome the trials and persecutions of this world, we will receive our reward and citizenship in Heaven. Jesus Christ paid the price for our admission, has prepared a place for us and is there waiting for us.

Reading the book of Revelation, the first time after I had accepted my short tenure on this earth opened my eyes. I gained a new understanding of the next stop on my journey, and a funny thing happened; I got excited about it. Read Chapter 21 if you want to share that excitement. John witnesses the Holy City, the glorious New Jerusalem, coming down out of Heaven. An angel shows John how this city was constructed from the walls, gates, and materials down to the 12 foundations made of precious stones. The angel who served as his tour guide even measured the size of the city. It's a detailed description of something we can only begin to imagine.

And, it is awesome. So awesome that we can't even begin to picture it. The warning is right there on the label. It's a "glory beyond comparison." The God who created our mind and imagination knew neither was big enough to contemplate the glory of Heaven let alone the New Jerusalem. The New Jerusalem, built for us as our inheritance, has the brilliance of a precious jewel according to the scriptures. It's a city of gold as pure as glass. It shines with the glory of God. It is so grand and so glorious that no human mind can conceive it. It is far beyond anything we have ever known. Take the most opulent castle, sanctuary or structure man has built. Multiply that by a million. Or, more. That's the New Jerusalem.

Remember the feeling standing at the south rim of the Grand Canyon? No photograph or painting does justice to that kind of grandeur. Remember walking along the edge of a La Jolla cliff and staring into the Pacific Ocean? No words adequately capture that moment. Remember looking over the tops of the Rocky Mountains from the summit of Pikes Peak? Those things we could imagine. Push all those images to the extreme edge of your comprehension. It's not quite enough to get your imagination all the way to the glory that is your eternal home.

There is room for all of us in this huge place. The New Jerusalem, according to John's vision, is constructed in the shape of a square. Each side is 1,400 miles long. That totals 2,000,000 square miles of incomparable riches. What an incredible home to imagine. Best of all, there is plenty of room for you and everyone you will ever meet.

And, it will be a great place to spend eternity. Better than the best vacation ever. Better than a day at the beach with no mosquitos. That warm day at the perfect temperature with no chance of getting a sunburn. The day the sand gives way to your feet and doesn't stick to your toes. The day the glass of sweet tea within easy reach never empties. And, after consuming all that tea, you never have to use the bathroom. Relaxing Jimmy Buffett songs play continuously that day. Heaven is even better. There will be no more tears, no more death nor mourning, crying or pain. *"Nothing impure will ever enter it, nor will anyone who does what is shameful or deceitful, but only those whose names are written in the Lamb's book of life."* (Revelation 21:27)

God and Jesus will live there, too. Right next door. The thrones of God and the Lamb (Jesus) will be right there within easy floating distance in this glorious city. We will see them face to face and live among them. We will be His people and He will be our God. There is no temple. God and Jesus are its temples. There is no need for the sun or electricity for light. The glory of God gives it light, and the Lamb is its lamp. There is no night there, and no being will ever close the gates. There will be no need for additional security.

Can you imagine seeing Jesus? Can you imagine looking directly into His loving eyes? Can you imagine the love and perfection that envelops you? Can you imagine kneeling at the feet of your Heavenly Father? I'm sure you've thanked them for the many blessings in your life. Can you even contemplate doing that again face to face? How do you express your appreciation for the sacrifice Jesus made? How do you say thank you to a father who sent his only son to die a violent and agonizing death for you? I can't quite picture it but I know it will happen somehow and the Father and the Son know my heart already. They know my every thought. They have numbered every hair on my head. There is nothing I could express that they don't already know. But I am looking forward to trying.

And, what is to become of us? We get an extreme makeover. Our bodies will be transformed to be like Jesus' glorious body. We will shine like the sun. We will be like the angels in Heaven. We will go from perishable to imperishable, from dishonor to glory, from weakness to power. Our natural bodies will be raised as a spiritual body. Best of all, we will be complete. We'll finish the transformation we experience here on Earth.

And, what will we do? We'll have some time on our hands as eternity is a long time. The first order of business will be taking a long look around and seeing what God has provided for us. We will see the truth through a new pair of eyes. Our job description is the same. We will continue serving God, but our service will be perfected. We will praise and worship God. We will reign with Him. What a great job description or a to-do list. What a great future we have. What a great hope.

Can you imagine? Can you imagine a God who loves us so much that He prepares this kind of life eternal for us?

Today, I no longer fear death. I'm looking forward to it. I have gone from abject fear to hopeful expectancy. It is our instinct to cling to life and survive at all cost but with eternity so grand waiting for us, how could you not want to shed the pain, the chemo side effects, and life's worries and make the move? I'm excited about eternal life in the New Jerusalem, and I can't wait to get there. It doesn't have to be tomorrow. I'll go when my mission here is finished. The hope of eternal life and the New Jerusalem will get me through a lot of hardships and help me endure the additional trials that accompany this earthly life. Once God's purpose for me has been fulfilled, I'll happily take the next step into eternity with Him.

The wisdom of knowing the short number of our living days includes a deeper understanding and appreciation of what happens after we die. Fully realizing the incredible gift of eternal life is exciting, comforting and the source of great hope. The closer this step is, the more you loosen the tight grip on this world and start looking ahead to eternal life with the Father and the Son. Every earthly sight you see and even the most thrilling experiences you may have pales in comparison to what lies ahead. When one weighs the challenges of day-to-day life, they lose their importance in the shadows of eternal life which is now within your grasp.

There is a grim side to all this talk of eternity. While God makes all things new in the New Jerusalem, he will wipe away the old earth. The earth we see is temporary, and everything in it will be gone. It will cease to exist. The Bible details the destruction of the earth and the suffering of those still alive in the last days. Those who don't believe, turn their backs or choose not to receive the gift of eternal life will be consigned to the fiery lake of burning sulfur. As believers, receivers and children of the Most High God, we will escape that fate and enjoy an eternal life of complete joy serving God. The others will not. No matter how good they seem or how well-intended they are or how many puppies they have saved, unless their names appear in the Book of Life, they are not getting into the New Jerusalem. They are doomed to an eternity separated from God. An eternity of pain and anguish.

Heaven is real. So is hell. So is the fiery lake. There is a clear fork in the road for us, and we choose which path we will take. My greatest fear is that there are people I love who won't experience the glory of eternal life. The thought of them traveling the wrong path, declining God's loving gift and spending eternity in the fiery lake is horrifying. It's a great motivator also. It is motivation to demonstrate God's light in my life. It is motivation to share what gives me hope. It is motivation to proclaim the joy and many benefits of believing in Jesus Christ, surrendering to Him and living a great adventure as a child of God. I'd sure like to know that my friends and family will also experience the joy of Christian life and the hope of glorious eternal life. I don't want to imagine them deceived by the temptations of this world and facing the fiery lake.

When life is short, I can't imagine anything more important than the assurance of salvation. I can't imagine anything more important than the assurance that eternal life is yours. Knowing who I am and whose I am is the greatest comfort and brings the complete peace that is so important to pressing on through this world. I cling to the promise of eternal life in the glorious New Jerusalem, and it gives me great hope.

I intensely appreciate the fact that God shared this vision of a glorious future. He documented it so well and gave all of us the same opportunity to study, to know and to accept this gracious gift.

Have you?

Chapter 7
Farewell Tour, Phase 2

Please excuse my strange sense of humor one more time. As the weeks passed, I started to get some visits from friends and family members. Usually, when we got together with folks living in other locations, we went to see them. Since the cancer diagnosis, they started to come to Texas to see us. I appreciated the visits and had a great time with the people I care about, and I labeled these visits Phase Two of The Farewell Tour. In Phase One, I was dealing with my mortality and saying goodbye to the people, events, and things that were important to me. In Phase Two, other people were coming here to say goodbye to me.

You may immediately disagree with my premise thinking that these are good folks with good intentions wanting to express their caring and concern for my welfare and not deserving of any satirical labeling. And, you would be 100% correct. But, I tend to go a few steps too far and put an ironic twist on things. Plus, these visits are unusual. While they were always possible and would be perfectly normal, this type of visit rarely happened.

I welcomed these visits and looked forward to them. It gave me a chance to tell people how I felt about them face-to-face. I could express how much they meant to me and how important our relationship has been. Hopefully, I had demonstrated that in one form or another over the years, but these visits gave me a chance to come right out and say it.

Expressing my feelings for people does not come naturally. I feel it, but I'm not that good at saying it. My siblings are spread out all over the country, and we see each other maybe once a year. My out-of-town friends are spread out as well, and we would see them occasionally when our travels brought us nearby. I'd meet with local friends when big events or work projects would bring us together. We would typically indulge in lighthearted conversations with lots of laughter and plenty of commentary on politics or current events. We'd rarely venture into the expression of feelings or delve deeply into heavy subjects.

When you don't have much time left, things change. When it might be the last time you see a person you care about, the conversation tends to go in a different direction. You aren't afraid to bring up much more important topics and those deep feelings come right to the surface.

Others feel the same way but don't always know how to express it. But the fact that they are here reaching out and making an effort means everything. It's the same for anyone in similar circumstances. One way or another, we'll communicate the love we have for each other. We may stumble over the words or fumble a few well-intended statements, but the meaning comes through loud and clear. Often through a laugh. Maybe through a tear. Mostly through a hug. Those tight embraces that you don't want to end are the best.

September 1, Day -286

The first Farewell Tour, Phase Two visit came from one of Cindy's closest friends. We were neighbors in Arizona, and she came all the way from Brooklyn to spend a few days with us. Lives, families, and careers pulled these good friends apart sending Cindy to Texas and her friend to New York. They kept in touch over the years, and it was an honor to have her visit. Her husband reached out with one of the first calls of support I received after the cancer diagnosis.

Was this a good time to tell Cindy about the revelation? Not sharing this dramatic event in my life wasn't sitting well. Was it time for me to man up and do the right thing? Was it time to give her the benefit of the doubt, tell her the story and let the chips fall where they may? Maybe Cindy could confide in her friend if I dropped the bomb before her arrival.

I don't think so. I convinced myself once again that sharing this news would ruin the visit. Cindy and her friend had plenty to talk about and stories to share without making it all about me. That's how I rationalized not confiding in my best friend this time. But the guilt was building, and my desire was building to share both the struggle and the triumph that had come from the revelation. The time would come soon.

As far to the right as you could place me on the political scale, you could put Cindy's friend on the left. In this day and age, it's hard to avoid any political conversations. And who wants to? They can be fun if you don't take them too personally. We couldn't find any issues we could agree on, but that didn't seem to matter. With the 800-pound cancer gorilla looming in the shadows, there wasn't much of a reason to try to convince the other that their point of view was misguided if not well intended. She was too polite to hurl any insults, and I wasn't about to say anything that might spoil the occasion. We came to the point where we would laugh at how far apart we were and agreed to disagree. Our relationship and the mutual expression of love, support and encouragement were more important than any petty political disagreement. Wouldn't it be refreshing if all of us could find that place?

How different the world would be if all of us had the wisdom of knowing the number of our years and were able to set our petty differences aside. How deep would you dig your heels and how many lines would you draw in the sand if you knew your time was short?

October 30, Day -227

The Farewell Tour, Phase 2 visits continued with a sibling reunion. My sister and two of my brothers arrived with spouses from three different cities and stayed at nearby hotels. Entertaining folks is easy in The Woodlands, Texas with so many dining, shopping and entertainment choices within walking distance. We don't have to tackle complicated transportation arrangements. We can meet somewhere, decide on a destination or activity and take a short stroll to get there.

We didn't wander far for the first awkward meeting. We gathered in the first place that could accommodate us, the lobby bar at their hotel. I had spoken many times on the phone and through text messaging with my family members, but this was the first face-to-face visit since the cancer diagnosis. My goal was to put a brave face on the circumstances. I wanted them to see that I had accepted those circumstances and was at peace so that they might be, too. There were many medical stories to tell that had those ironic twists to them and I had a host of new experiences to share. I was between chemotherapy cycles, so I felt pretty good and I wanted them to see that I wasn't on my deathbed yet.

They wanted to be encouraging, show their support and see for themselves exactly how I was doing. Our phone conversations before this visit wouldn't reveal anything other than an upbeat approach to dealing with some tough medical issues leaving many unanswered questions. The medical explanations and descriptions of treatments were complicated, and each sibling had their missing details. They wanted to express their support for Cindy as well. They could imagine the hard work of a caregiver and the pain of potentially losing a spouse. Their encouragement and offers of assistance would be more than welcome.

This new world of chemotherapy treatments and medications included more frequent trips to the bathroom. When that inevitable time came, I excused myself and walked down the hallway to the men's room. Poor Cindy. As soon as I was safely out of earshot, they pounced with questions.

"How is he <u>really</u> doing?" my brother asked. "What is he not telling us?"

Cindy bravely fought back the tears that always linger just below the surface and addressed all the questions until I returned to the table. We'd have to get used to that. It happens every time we meet with people.

I loved playing tour guide to our little town during the three-day visit. They had little interest in activities like movies or dining in fancy places but wanted to find unique places to congregate and have conversations. We found ourselves outdoors one evening gathered around a fire pit with one of those board games meant to get people talking and telling stories. With the water taxis floating down the Waterway and the setting sun in the background, we had a great time trying to outdo each other with a more outlandish point of view or perspective on a social dilemma. The game provided some relief from talking about my health issues allowing me to have some simple fun with people I loved. Like the old days.

There was plenty of time for individual conversations as well. There were opportunities to speak as couples or individuals where subjects could get a little deeper or a little more personal. I was ready and willing to go as deep or as personal as they wanted to go. I confess going deep myself whenever I would see an opportunity. If I had a shot, I'd take it. I'd start a conversation about my favorite topics such as faith, life after death, the meaning of life and our purpose here on earth. Aren't those everyone's favorite topics? These were uncomfortable conversations for some, but they were important to me. What was the point in holding anything back? What was the point of small talk? Don't worry; I didn't push them too far. I got pretty good at reading the room and would back off if I saw folks squirm. I didn't want these welcome visitors to feel anxious or awkward, but I did want them to think about what they would do if they had a few months or years to live. I wanted them to find themselves in the place where I was, appreciating the simple joys of life and letting go of some of those burdens that cause us to miss so many of life's true pleasures.

The wisdom revealed in knowing the number of your years creates a desire for stronger and deeper relationships. Not only do people treat you differently but you also treat them differently. There are no chance encounters. No random meetings. Each time you cross paths with someone it opens a new door. Each contact is an opportunity to let God's light shine brightly and to display God's love by doing something good for the people you meet. I found myself caring so much more deeply about people and placing a much higher value on the time spent with them. I didn't want to waste a single moment.

My sister cried first when it came time to say goodbye at the airport. I had a hard time trying to maintain my composure, but somewhere deep down inside there was some additional peace that helped me stand tall through what could be the last hugs and handshakes. When your days are numbered, goodbyes become a lot more difficult.

November 30, Day -196

Not long after the visit from my sister and brothers I got a visit from my youngest daughter and her family. I thought I had said goodbye to them for the last time 11 months ago in Phase One of The Farewell Tour. This visit was a "bonus" in Phase Two and certainly a blessing. The adoration for these kids, four of them now, continued strong and kept growing deeper.

This visit was a first. It was so much easier and much less expensive for Cindy and me to jump on a plane and head for Southern California than for two adults and four young children to fly to Texas. But, what a treat. This visit was the first opportunity to show off our downsized and maintenance free walking lifestyle and to spend time with the grandchildren on our home turf. We had always talked about how the kids would enjoy the wildlife in the area. Egrets were familiar sights fishing in the Waterway. Ducks, turtles, and fish were also plentiful and easy to find and feed. The Woodlands is also home to a mounted patrol, so horses were a common sight plodding down the city streets. Water taxis and trolley cars transported visitors from place to place. These would be unusual sights for them, and we couldn't wait to see how the girls would react.

Their visit came early in the holiday season. The Woodlands went all out for the holidays, and the town was fully wrapped with multicolored lights, tall Christmas trees, and holiday decorations. Market Street, the "town square" of The Woodlands, hosted musical light shows, carriage rides and even made sure that artificial snow filled the night sky on the weekends. We knew the girls would love it and we couldn't wait to watch them take it all in.

The grandchildren had no idea I had a terminal illness. We focused every moment with them on sharing experiences and exploring the area. There would be no discussion of how I felt or taking it easy because Papa might not be up to any vigorous exercise. I still had plenty of energy assisted by the adrenaline boost from seeing the girls. While I had lost a step or two, I was sure they wouldn't notice. And, Vidaza had been kind to my hairline, so there were no visible signs of illness. There would be nothing but wholesome family adventures and new experiences through the eyes of these beautiful kids. They were blissfully unaware of the real reason for the trip.

The more in-depth conversations with my daughter and son-in-law took place in stolen moments away from the girls. They were few in number but enough to communicate that I was okay. I was okay physically at that time. I was okay mentally and spiritually. I was at peace. I went out of my way to demonstrate the fact that I was okay so that they would be okay. I wanted them to feel the same peace that I had. We made sure there was enough time for them to ask grown-up questions, touch home base and express their support and encouragement.

The girls took turns spending the night with Grammy and Papa. We enjoyed spending time with them as a group, but the one on one time was priceless. An overnight stay always led to an early morning outing with their grandfather.

"Do you want to sneak out and a donut?" I asked knowing the answer. No child can refuse that offer.

We'd whisper to each other as we hurried into some walking clothes and a light jacket and tip-toed out the door. We took the long way to the grocery store which included an exploration of the many Waterway adventures, watching for baby ducklings and checking to see if the turtle eggs had hatched. We'd visit the parks and check in on the Koi with names like Sunshine, Blueberry, Bones, Chicken Pox and Clown Nose. These adventures were not guided tours. Think of a child on the loose freely exploring a new and exciting place with an "enabler" and protector in close pursuit. I always made sure we stopped along the way and let the kids do those little things that harried parents don't have time for in their busy schedules.

I love these little adventures. It's part of what makes being a grandparent so much fun and rewarding. But my time is limited, and my opportunities are few. My short-timer attitude makes the experience so much different. So much deeper. So much better. If you doubt the likelihood that it will ever happen again, you savor every moment of the experience. You thank God for each minute that you have with them. You stretch it out as long as possible. You have as much fun as you can. You make the experience unforgettable for you and the child. You are entirely in the moment.

If many such visits are likely, each one loses its significance. You might miss some of the fun. You might not have as much patience. There will always be another day. Another visit. Another experience. The danger of that kind of perspective is that soon they will move on. The kids will grow up. School starts. They develop other interests. They get busy. The moment has passed you by.

If you are fortunate enough to have dozens of such experiences, enjoy each one to the fullest. These are the most important things in this life. Don't let a single one slip through your fingers.

Many benefits accompany a cancer diagnosis. This visit from my grandchildren was one of them. These adventures would never have happened if I didn't have bone marrow cancer. Something would invariably arise to cause a postponement. There would always be an excellent reason not to make such an arduous trip. When time is short, a lot of those excuses fall by the wayside. If it is ever going to happen, it has to happen now. I am most grateful for that.

Close friends of over 40 years came for a visit a few months later. We met this special couple when we were young and stayed connected through four decades of successes, failures, jobs, marriages (he was in my wedding party), children and grandchildren. We kept in touch through the up times and the down times. The seasons of plenty and the seasons of lack. This welcome visit was due directly to the cancer diagnosis. During their stay in

The Woodlands, we shared family updates, jokes, political perspectives and attended a Tom Petty concert at the nearby Cynthia Woods Mitchell Pavilion, one of the most successful outdoor concert venues in the country. We stopped by Target on the way to pick up some rain ponchos determined not to let an 80% chance of showers spoil our evening. The music didn't stop when the rain started to fall, and we kept our chairs while others ran for the exits. That was a good decision. We knew my days were numbered but had no idea that Tom Petty's days were numbered as well.

These delightful people are empty nesters like us in a similar stage of life, and there is no shortage of conversation topics. We savored every moment. We didn't waste one second.

Here we are again with another painful goodbye. The assurance that I had squeezed every good moment out of the time I had made it a little easier. Cindy and I were so grateful for their visit that it was hard to be too sad when it was time for them to go. We compressed a hundred such visits into a couple of productive days. We had to.

I am more convinced than ever that this is the best way to live your life whether you have a terminal illness or not. If you can get to that place where you honestly believe that time is short and each encounter could be your last, a beautiful world begins to unfold where you spend your time and put your effort into maximizing every experience. Each one of those experiences deepens and become much more meaningful. You embrace your friends more tightly and make the most of each moment. You begin to see things differently recognizing blessings in places where you had never seen them before. You catch a glimpse of God's grace and might and love in almost everything you encounter.

What a beautiful way to live! I am so grateful that God revealed it to me, allowed me to live into that wisdom for a few years and gave me the opportunity to share it with you.

Chapter 8

Preparation for Transplant

Time passes quickly when it is in such short supply. It has been 18 months since the revelation and 12 months since the cancer diagnosis. I had endured 91 chemotherapy treatments and had adapted to this cyclical world of sickness and health. One week of the nasty flu and hangover symptoms were followed by three weeks of recovery every month. Each series of treatments brought new side effects, and it seemed to take longer to bounce back from each following cycle. Recovery would be a little less complete each time. It was taking a toll on my body and speeding up the aging process to the point where I could almost feel it. It seemed like I had aged about 12 years in the past 12 months. I maintained a schedule of weight training and running though the weights were lighter and the miles were fewer.

Vidaza, the primary chemotherapy drug used to control the cancerous stem cells in Myelodysplastic Syndrome cases can keep blast counts low for a couple of years, but for most patients, the disease stops responding after about 12 months. How long would it work for me? It depends. Scientists are studying new drugs, but only Vidaza and its cousin Dacogen are FDA approved. Once Vidaza runs its course, a patient has only one option. The long shot. The "Hail Mary" pass. The Stem Cell Transplant.

At about the same time as chemotherapy begins, the search for a potential stem cell donor begins. It's a long lead time item and can take months to locate a donor. Siblings are always the best candidates for donation and are most likely to be a full match. I have four siblings, and I was sure I'd have a couple of options. However, only one was a full match. Two siblings got half way there with 50% matches. One was not a match at all. I harbor the possibility that my youngest brother sent someone else's blood. But, no harm no foul since my oldest brother was a 100% match. Plus, he was in the best physical condition. He worked out regularly, ate well, didn't smoke and led a pretty healthy lifestyle. If you lined up my four siblings, he would be your first choice, and he would have an easier time with the donation process.

February 1, Day -133

A few months after the testing, I got a call from my healthy brother Mike.

"Hey, big boy!" Mike said in his usual upbeat greeting, but his tone changed quickly. "I got some news today."

When his voice cracked, I knew the next sentence was not going to be good. It came a couple of seconds later and each word sounded painful.

"I can't… donate… my stem cells."

The declaration landed like a one-two punch. The first punch was hearing that the matching stem cells I counted on were gone. I blocked that punch shifting immediately to my concern for Mike. Something was wrong, and he wasn't well. He contracted a disease of his own that disqualified him as a donor. I wanted to find out more about his health, but he wanted to talk about mine.

Mike took pride in the idea of being my liberator. He was a hero is coming to the rescue of an ailing brother. Now, he felt helpless letting me down. I assured him that I'd be able to find an unrelated donor. I cited the fact that our tissue type was one of the easiest to match. I hoped it was true and that things would turn out that way.

When I asked about his health, he assured me that everything would be okay. There were medications and treatments that would get him back on his feet.

I passed that bombshell along to Dr. Kornblau at my next exam.

"That's not going to work," he said with a look of serious business on his face.

He spun a half turn to the left in his exam room chair and rolled over to the computer desk without missing a beat. He sent that news flash to the stem cell department. But there was a bright side. He let me know that while stem cells from a related donor resulted in a lower chance of rejection, studies showed a higher chance of relapse after the transplant. Stem cells from an unrelated donor came with a higher chance of rejection but a lower incidence of relapse. I took some good notes and made sure my generous ailing brother knew those statistics.

Dr. Kornblau's email got the ball rolling. The transplant team submitted my name and tissue type to an international donor registry called "Be The Match." Technicians compared my tissue type to samples received from potential donors around the world to find the closest match possible.

Researchers have identified 14 markers to match tissue types. Ten are considered high priority markers. The more markers that line up, the better the match with the least amount of rejection.

After a couple of months, the good news arrived. A potential donor, a 33-year-old male, had been located in Western Europe. That's all they would tell me. The identities of the donor and recipient are a well-kept secret for two years. I could probably get the recipe for Coca-Cola or Kentucky Fried Chicken easier than the name of the stem cell donor. If both parties agree, the registry reveals their identities after the two-year waiting period.

Why Western Europe? The nurse coordinating the donor search showed no surprise that the donor lived halfway across the globe. She said a much higher percentage of the population of Europe and other countries register as potential donors than people in the United States. European donors are not uncommon at all. Stem cell research and the benefits of stem cell transplants are well known in Europe but not common knowledge in America. We'll have to change that! We can start with a shameless plug for the "Be The Match" organization and their website, www.bethematch.org. I've included more information on "Be The Match" and how to register in the appendix section of this book.

March 15, Day -91

The researchers had identified a potential donor and the time had come to consider a transplant. The Vidaza was losing its punch, and the percentage of cancerous stem cells was on the rise. During a monthly visit to MD Anderson and a consultation with my doctor, he carefully introduced the option as if he were placing an expensive vase on the table for us to appraise. We had discussed this vase several times, and I was fully aware of its value and fragile nature. Doc always put the transplant option on the back burner and considered it an ace in the hole and would play it only if he had to. The fact that he offered it as a possibility now meant he believed I was running out of options and things could easily take a turn for the worst. The greatest fear was an increase in the blast count, the percentage of cancerous stem cells to normal stem cells in my bone marrow, and a progression to Acute Myeloid Leukemia.

A Stem Cell Transplant is not an easy procedure to consider. It is a miraculous potential cure but comes with a high level of risk.

Up to 30% of those who undergo a transplant don't survive it. And, it only works 50% of the time. It's a harrowing experience and requires two years to recover. I told myself that MD Anderson statistics would probably be better than national averages since they were among the world's finest facilities, had the best doctors and complete 900 such transplants every year.

I reasoned with myself over the last 12 months that if or when the time came, I'd have a few advantages. I was a little younger and in better physical condition than most who undergo this procedure and my "do or die" attitude would be helpful. That is literally true in this case. I may sail right through this thing, or I may die trying. As with everything else in my world, it depends.

Dr. Kornblau described the procedure again along with the risks. He was purposeful in avoiding a specific recommendation stating that this was my decision. Despite my best efforts to pin him down, he would not declare a professional or personal opinion. I had to find that answer in his eyes, his mannerisms and his body language. I am not a good poker player, but I think I caught a tell. His eyes conveyed the belief that his best chance of a successful outcome was to do it now rather than wait any longer.

Despite my fear of the process I couldn't help but agree. I wasn't getting any younger, any healthier or any more handsome. The longer I waited the harder the procedure would be.

Cindy leaned towards taking the chance, but she fell short of representing a definitive opinion. She left it to me after, once again, pledging her full back up and support. She was in as deep as I was since she would have to shoulder the difficult role of caregiver and would have to place her life on hold while helping me through this demanding process. A person wouldn't even be considered for transplant without a 24 hour a day caregiver.

What would you do? Would you take the chance? Would you stay the course and live out the rest of your days as you had been? Was the possibility of a "cure" worth the risk of death or the pain of the transplant procedure? Would a few more years be worth the toll the transplant would take on your body and mind?

I prayed. Boy, did I pray. I didn't want even to consider gathering the troops and going into this battle without first inquiring of the Lord.

"Lord, what is your will? What would you have me do?"

I couldn't fight this battle on my own. I couldn't depend on my own strength, my own perseverance or my own determination. That kind of pride or confidence had left me long ago. Why even approach such a risky procedure without the full backing of a powerful and loving God?

Prayers continued for several days. Cindy and I prayed together and separately for an answer. Should the transplant be undertaken? Is now the time? Is this the place? Is there another path I should be considering?

The answer came swiftly, clearly and again with few words. God revealed that it didn't matter what decision I made. He reminded me that He was bigger than anything I faced. My God was bigger than cancer, transplants or any circumstances I could encounter.

It seemed as if I had stepped into a clearing after a long trek through the woods. A few moments ago I had a question. I now had the answer as if deciphering a code that had eluded me for quite some time. The outcome would be the same no matter which path I chose. God was here, He was in control, and He had me in the palm of His hand.

A person could interpret that in one of two ways. Don't be afraid of the transplant. Or, there is no need for the transplant. After all, the outcome would be the same. God would bring me to the same place no matter which path I chose.

The answer required another decision. Would you avail yourself to the best medicine, procedures, and facilities on earth?

Or, would you shun the transplant and let the chips fall where they may? Logic may point to the medical solution. Faith may point to God's infinite healing power and a spiritual solution.

I don't know if I made the right decision but the thought that it didn't matter provided some relief. I took the road leading to the transplant keeping an option open that a miracle could happen along the way. I would listen for an inner conviction that I had come to appreciate. That conviction would signal a coming crash and illuminate the correction that was needed. The team was busy making plans, preparations were underway, and momentum was building. I never felt a conviction or had the sense that I was taking the wrong path. I felt God's active presence. I was not alone. He was with me. He would fight the battle, and the outcome was certain.

Cindy fully supported the plan. Dr. Kornblau didn't tip his hand when we presented the decision, but after another read of his body language, I was sure he thought we had chosen the right path.

Here we go.

The transplant team wasted no time setting the hospital admission date. An intense dosage of chemotherapy would be administered the first four days to utterly destroy my existing bone marrow and all the cancerous stem cells in it. After a couple of days to recover and flush the chemotherapy drugs out of my system, the new donor stem cells would be infused into my bloodstream to replace the old cells and rebuild the bone marrow. Sounds simple enough. What could possibly go wrong?

The stem cell infusion isn't all that intricate and resembles a blood transfusion. It's the complications from the chemotherapy and rejection of the foreign stem cells that cause all the problems. These complications occur in different ways and different levels of intensity for each person. The doctors tell you that something will go haywire. They just can't predict what that will be or its level of intensity. The success of the transplant will depend on how quickly they can identify problems and how effectively they can treat them. MD Anderson had completed thousands of stem cell transplants and had seen even more complications. Mine could hardly be unique or a surprise. That's reassuring, right?

It takes about 30 days to go to the brink and back. A month-long hospital stay is required to complete the preparative chemotherapy, transplant the stem cells and treat any of the issues that occur afterward. Then, you have to plan on spending another two months within 15 minutes of the MD Anderson emergency room to get there quickly should a problem develop. You're not out of the woods in 90 days, but usually, the most serious problems would occur in that time frame. Most relapses occur in the first year. If two years pass with no serious issues, a stem cell transplant patient can anticipate a normal life expectancy.

What? Normal life expectancy? Me? Is that possible? How does that square with God's revelation that he is calling me home soon? I had wrapped my mind around the fact that my time on earth was short. Most likely I'd die of bone marrow cancer within three to five years of the diagnosis. I had gone from the thought that I could die at any moment to the notion that I might have a few years to live. I couldn't let myself even imagine the possibility that I could ever again have a normal life expectancy.

And, God didn't say that. He didn't say that if I conquered MDS that I would have a normal life expectancy. God made it clear that the opposite was true. The medical "cure" didn't matter. He would fulfill His good purpose either way.

Did God ever change His mind? Is there a biblical precedent for such a notion? God listened to Moses and relented from destroying the rebellious Israelites in the desert. Could that apply to me? What if someone like Moses would intercede on my behalf? Many good people were praying for me. Would God act on their intercession? Would God grant me a few more years if it fulfilled His purpose and my vessel could be used to accomplish His will?

The prophet Ezekiel asked God not to make him defile himself with a fire fueled by human waste. Could God give me a similar change of instructions as detailed in the 4th chapter of Ezekiel?

I happened to be reading the Old Testament a few months before the transplant. And a particular series of verses happened to leap from the pages of 2 Kings in chapters 18, 19 and 20. It's the story of Hezekiah, King of Judah. Hezekiah was one of the good kings putting his faith in God and straightening out the mess left by his evil-doing father Ahaz. His little kingdom prospered even though much larger and more powerful enemies surrounded it.

Hezekiah fell sick from a boil and was near death. He got a visit from Isaiah the prophet with a message from the Lord telling him to set his house in order because he would surely die.

Hezekiah wept bitterly after an appeal to God which is considered one of the great prayers of the Old Testament. God stopped Isaiah before he could even get out of the building to go back and tell Hezekiah that his prayers were heard, his tears were recognized, and he would be healed. God would add 15 years to Hezekiah's life and protect Judah from an Assyrian assault from the north.

I zoomed in on another essential part of the story and the next step in the healing process. Isaiah applied a treatment to the boil to facilitate the healing and Hezekiah's recovery. Why was the treatment needed? In this case, there was no immediate or spontaneous cure. Some action had occurred on the part of Isaiah the prophet and Hezekiah the king to complete the healing. Could a transplant serve the same purpose as Hezekiah's boil treatment? Should I have more skin in the game?

The parallels were striking to me. God sent a message to Hezekiah saying that he was going to die. After hearing Hezekiah's appeal, God used a medical procedure to heal him.

Could this story apply to me? Could history repeat itself? Could God heal my cancer and give me 15 more years after saying he was calling me home soon? Would God respond to my cries and genuine repentance? Is it possible that the revelation had nothing to do with the cancer I was fighting? Maybe I'd be called home soon regardless of any medical treatment I had.

I held on to the possibility that if God was using cancer to bring me home soon, that He could grant me a 15-year extension. He had done similar things before.

These were some of the thoughts and questions lurking in my mind as I went into the most grueling physical challenge of my life. I had no answers. I had no certainty. But I did have a deep well of faith and trust in a loving and present God.

I was sure, however, that I should always see my days as numbered. I should live my life one day at a time. I should make no long-term plans. I must depend on God and not myself, doctors or medical procedures. I should convey the wisdom of numbered years to other people. I should be a living example and explain the benefits of such a perspective to anyone who would listen.

In retrospect, God wasn't changing His mind. He was changing me. He was transforming me and preparing me for the next phase of my life no matter how long or how short that life may be.

May 22, Day -23

Two weeks before admission day, Cindy and I returned to MD Anderson for a full battery of physical tests to make sure my body could withstand the chemotherapy and stem cell infusion. I aced the lung function test, and a series of ultrasounds showed that my internal organs were in good shape. My eyes checked out a little dry but okay. The dental division recommended a root canal before the transplant to clean up some decay they had spotted that might flare up and cause some problems. A root canal right before a stem cell transplant? Seriously? That's asking a bit too much don't you think? After talking with the doctor, I decided to take my chances and forgo the root canal.

How much chemotherapy could I take? Yes, there is a test for that. It involved two 12-hour days where I was infused with a small amount of the primary drug Busulfan and monitored every 15 minutes to see how my body reacted. It wasn't painful, just a long, tough day. I aced that test, too, and qualified for the full standard dosage. Lucky me.

May 24, Day -21

One final procedure closed any possible escape hatch. I was fitted with my own brand new central venous catheter, or CVC to make it easier to administer drugs and medications. No need to swallow pills or take shots or search for veins in your arm to insert an IV line. The CVC line, about a foot in length, was inserted directly into my subclavian vein just under the right collarbone to get the fluids directly into my bloodstream near the heart.

A small plastic disc about the size of a quarter is stitched into the skin and holds the lines in place. I would sport three tubes called lumens about four inches in length hanging from the right side of my upper chest. Tubes are connected to those lumens to administer drugs or fluids and draw blood. A bandage covers the spot where the main tube disappears right into the skin. I'll spare you the details of the installation process. I'll just say it's uncomfortable but there large quantities of Lidocaine used to minimize the pain. At this point, I'd been stuck, prodded, probed and injected enough that by comparison, the procedure wasn't all that tough. Besides, this would reveal itself as one of the least painful aspects of the stem cell transplant. I did wonder, however, how were they going to take this thing out?

With these lumens hanging from my chest, I know I'm a stem cell transplant patient. It's on now.

Cindy, me and my brand-new lumens attended a pre-admission stem cell transplant class that would provide the final overview of what we could expect and how we might mentally prepare for the procedure. In a matter of fact style, one of the slides stated that the IV connection (via my shiny new lumens) would be in place for the entire 30-day hospital stay. No breaks. Therefore, I'd have to come up with shirts I could put on and remove without disrupting the IV line(s).

There were a lot of surprises like that. Repeated punches in the gut with varying intensity. The 24 hours 7 day a week IV line surprise was one of the easy ones. The duration (forever) of the initial chemotherapy plan was the granddaddy of them all and provided the biggest bad surprise to date. Hopefully, a successful transplant would alleviate the need for any more of those nasty monthly chemotherapy treatments.

June 7, Day -7

Admission day had finally arrived. God had not closed this door for me even though I was looking for it. My antenna was up and receptive to any feeling of conviction or any sign that I shouldn't move forward. I didn't feel one or see one. It was go time. Time to return to MD Anderson for a final doctor's appointment allowing Dr. Kornblau to give me one last exam before I was to take the short walk to the hospital and admission for my 30-day stay.

Don't you know that when you take your car into the shop, it stops making that noise that was so annoying before you made the appointment? In the same way, I was feeling pretty good despite all the tests and trying to get used to these tubes hanging out of my chest. My most recent lab results looked good, too. Key blood counts were up. The last bone marrow biopsy showed considerable improvement.

"Do you really think I need this transplant?" I asked. I was only half joking. "My numbers are excellent and I'm feeling good. Looks like I've been healed."

I seemed to catch a slight trace of hesitation on his part, but he didn't change his mind or reverse course. He jokingly responded that my last chance to bail out was before the intense chemotherapy treatments were administered in a couple of days.

"After that," he said, "the rocket has been launched."

There would be no turning back.

Now is the time to tell Cindy about the revelation don't you think? Here we are barreling down this bumpy path with unknown twists and turns. On this ride, you never know where it is going or if you would be in the car when it pulled back in the station. With the considerable risk involved, I should undoubtedly bite the bullet, put my fears aside, have the conversation and walk hand in hand into this great unknown. But it still didn't feel right. How could I add this burden to the anxieties she was already experiencing? How could I add more uncertainty to the most challenging time of our lives? I had the time to process the revelation and get my arms around it. Cindy wouldn't have that kind of time.

You guessed it. I caved. I couldn't do it. I did not share the revelation but told myself if I survived the transplant, we'd have that conversation. She should know. She should know everything. I should give her the respect and opportunity to deal with the news good or bad. It would not be pleasant, but I needed to have faith that she would be able to process it and work it out.

Carrying the secret with me, I swallowed hard, took a deep breath, glanced towards the Heavens and made my way to the admissions desk.

We made one more stop on the way. MD Anderson had a hair salon on the 6th floor, and since I'd be losing all my hair in a week or two anyway, Cindy and I stopped in to mark this occasion with a ceremonial buzz cut. Let's take the hair off now before it starts coming out in clumps later.

There were a couple of people ahead of me in line. Some folks were there for real styling of regrown hair. Others were doing what we were doing and proactively removing whatever hair they had left.

The man who walked in behind me was one of those proactive guys carrying an air of defiance. He was going to strike first in a battle between his active outdoor past and a disease trying to take it from him.

A stem cell transplant is a real act of defiance. It's the line in the sand. After giving up so much of yourself to insatiable cancer, the transplant was like bringing out the big guns. It was going nuclear in a gutsy last stand.

That's the same troubled feeling I harbored. I recognized it right away in this guy named Jim mixed with some engaging if not biting sarcasm and a dry sense of humor.

Jim dressed like an athlete warming up for a playoff game in a sweat suit and tennis shoes. He wore his uniform under a jacket ready to be revealed at game time. This haircut was part of the warm-up ritual. He knew that playing this game would cost him his hair and he didn't want to give his opponent the satisfaction of seeing it fall out. He would shave it in a preemptive strike that would signal his willingness to see this battle through to the end.

"Take my hair," Jim seemed to say. "I don't need it. But I'll fight to the death for the health I have left."

I wanted to be Jim's teammate and his friend. I wanted to join forces and fight cancer with him. He looked like my other friends who had helped me win other battles. He was just past working age with a few pounds to spare. I could use his help, and I knew he could use mine. The nerves he wore on his sleeves were at war with his sarcasm, and it sucked me into the battle. It brought my own sarcasm to the surface to reinforce his. I also had to up my witty quip-trading game since we were using humor to disguise the fact that we were both peeking nervously over the edge of a rugged cliff.

Neither one of us wanted to be here. Yet, here we stood ready to take a high dive into the same turbulent waters hoping we had the strength to swim through a strong current that would take us to places unknown. The jump didn't seem as treacherous with someone else to jump with you.

Jim's wife Coleen took a seat in a sitting room chair across the small waiting area where we could see the styling taking place a few feet away. Jim sat down right next to me and started the conversation.

"You getting a haircut?" he asked without any fanfare.

I told him I was in for a buzz cut.

"Me, too," was his reply. "You getting some chemo?" He pressed.

I described the chemo plan, the predicted hair loss, and my upcoming stem cell transplant.

"Me, too," he said. "I'm checking in right after this."

In the next few minutes, we became teammates. We exchanged diagnoses and short stories about how we wound up in this place at this time. I described my MDS. He described his Myelofibrosis. We were both throwing the Hail Mary pass and today was admission day, game day. The official transplant day was in exactly one week for both of us. We became fast friends and swapped contact information. It would be good for both of us to talk about this journey with someone who understood it perfectly. Someone who is going through the same procedure. Each of us had a new ally in this battle.

I went for the #1 setting on the clippers. My new friend Jim went for a complete head shave. Justine, the stylist, understood our situation. She laughed with us and put up with our jokes about how handsome we were and that we should have shaved our heads years ago. Our wives played along rolling their eyes and shaking their heads. What a blessing to make a few friends, find a teammate, have some fun and let off a little steam at such a serious time.

Was meeting Jim a coincidence? Maybe not.

We bumped into Jim and Coleen again downstairs in the hospital lobby. They had checked in, received their room assignment on the 17th floor and sat with their suitcases waiting a few more minutes as their room was going through its final inspections.

I followed his lead, walked through the lobby and found the check-in desk off in a corner by itself. It looked more like a concierge desk with only one person working and no lines. I leaned in and asked for a room on the 17th floor. I received a friendly smile but no compliance. Jim got the last one. Cindy and I were informed that we would spend the next 30 days on the 18th floor and our room would take another couple of hours to prepare. That was bad news and an obstacle to developing this new relationship. Patients were not allowed to leave their floors for the duration of their stays.

"I'll see you in a month," Jim said as he and Coleen stood and headed for the elevator.

"Or, before," I replied, confident that I would find the exceptions to the rule.

I didn't get a key, just a room assignment and directions to our little one-room studio on the 18th floor. That room full of medical equipment would be home sweet home for the next 30 days.

I walked in with a defiant little swagger. I didn't know how I would walk out, if at all.

Chapter 9
Stem Cell Transplant

Still feeling good, I took the express elevator up to the 18th floor then followed the signs to our suite. I tried not to look in the open doors of other suites we passed along the way, but I wanted to see how those occupants looked. Were they happy? Were they in pain? Did they have any energy? Were they doing anything? The rooms we passed represented all those circumstances, but they mostly showed signs of epic struggles. The door to room 1840 was open, so we stepped right in and checked out the furnishings like we would in any hotel room. I walked around the little studio opening the drawers, adjusting the small TV, inspecting the bathroom, checking out the view and testing the twin size hospital bed with a bounce or two.

The nicely furnished room has plenty of space, but when you cram in all the medical equipment, it shrinks considerably. This room exceeded our expectations and would compare favorably to a nice hotel with modern wood tones on the walls and floors that offset the neutral colors and sterile disinfected surfaces.

Walking into a typical hotel room, you tend to take over the space making it yours for a short period. This room seemed to push back as if to say, "*I've seen tougher men than you*" and "*you'll do things on my terms.*" Somehow, we'd have to make peace and work together for the next few weeks. We struck a deal where I agreed to be a thoughtful tenant and keep the place tidy. In exchange, the room would keep an eye on me and shelter me. There were no guarantees beyond that. When the treatments began, I was on my own. When pushed beyond my limits, the room would not come to my rescue. When my faith was tested, it was all me and my Creator. When the pain became intolerable, I'd have to dig in. I had no choice but to agree to those terms.

I kept looking back at the oversized door. There was one way in this room and only one way out. That imposing door would determine who came and went. Two linebackers in full pads could walk through that door shoulder to shoulder. It was thick enough to seal the room from the commotion in the hallway. It was big enough to get the bed and medical equipment in and out in a hurry or allow a team of doctors to rush in at the same time. The floor flowed seamlessly from the hallway into the room with no threshold to impede the progress.

Inside the room, it was down to business. No rugs, table lamps, plants or curtains. Any surface that could harbor a germ had been removed. Hospital staff could clean this room easily and quickly, and no bacteria had a chance at survival. I hoped my chances would be better.

The far corner of the room would become Cindy's corner with a small leather-like couch and a pullout extension that provided a little extra sleeping area. If she bent her legs and pulled her knees close to her chest, her feet wouldn't hang off the edge of the couch. At least the smooth surfaces would be easy to clean. She had every right to complain but flashed a polite grin instead and began to stack some of her things on the right side as if to say she could make it work. She acknowledged the lack of space but expressed her relief that she had a place to sleep and that we were able to share the same room.

Natural light found its way in through a small poster-sized window next to Cindy's corner. Other than the TV bolted to the wall, the view to the south was my connection to the outside world. From the height of the 18th floor, I could look down on the massive NRG Stadium a mile or so away. If I fully extended my neck and twisted it slightly to the right, I could see the sunset over the tall medical center buildings. My gaze shifted quickly to the left and locked on a medical helicopter. It flew in at eye level descending to a helipad on the 10th floor of the building next door. The cool factor of witnessing the landing sobered quickly as the medical team rushed out to wheel the passenger to the emergency room ducking from the blades that continued circling. This person needed the most drastic measures with no time to waste.

There were two such helipads within view, and I would witness hundreds of landings and takeoffs from all angles at all hours of the day and night.

Jim wound up on the 17th floor in a room about the same size and similarly furnished. I texted him immediately telling him how grateful we should be that we had such spacious rooms with oversized picture windows and plush king beds.

Jim: View is pretty good. I think I'm looking east. Small window. I got the master bath and a sofa. How about you?

Marc: Really? On the 18th floor there are huge picture windows, a master bath, sitting area and a king size bed.

Jim took my text at face value and wondered if he drew the short straw. I fessed up to the slight but intentional exaggeration on my part, and it was the last time he took one of my text messages seriously. Texting served as our primary form of communication, meager attempts at humor, and a lifeline when we needed one.

Following instructions, we brought a few changes of loose-fitting casual clothes that fit perfectly in the small built-in drawers.

I brought three small items to put my stamp on this space. I placed a 12-inch desktop cross on a shelf in the front part of the room. I leaned a picture of the starting line of the Conoco Phillips Rodeo Run 10k on a table reminding me of my goal to run that race eight months after the transplant.

The most important contribution to the decor of the hospital room was an 8x10 framed Bible verse from 2 Corinthians 4:17-18. *"For our light and momentary troubles are achieving for us an eternal glory that far outweighs them all. So we fix our eyes not on what is seen, but what is unseen, since what is seen is temporary, but what is unseen is eternal."* I hung that picture on the wall with Command Strips when no one was looking. I figured I'd apologize if I needed to rather than ask for permission to attach it to the wall. It took its place in the most visible spot in the room so that I could see it from the bed and remember that no matter how difficult this challenge would be, it was temporary. It would serve as a great reminder to look past the painful physical world around me and focus my attention on more peaceful spiritual matters. This prominent position would also draw the attention of any visitor and prove to be a great conversation starter.

A cheery nurse bounced through that imposing door and extended her hand.

"My name is Rosie," she said. The name fit her well. "We're going to take good care of you. What do you think of your new home?"

She took us on a short tour of the room and its various functions and equipment lingering in the bathroom where she detailed the importance of measuring everything going in and out of the body. The medical team would measure what went in. I had to measure what went out. Two urinals with measuring scales on the sides sat conveniently near the toilet that had a unique faucet for rinsing them. I was to post all measurements on the whiteboard near the big front door.

Rosie also had the task of connecting one of the lumens dangling from my chest to the fluids that would drip into my system continuously through my hospital stay. From the pre-admission class, I knew what to expect. Once connected, there would be no separation from the fluids or the rolling tree that held the bags. And no relief from the noise made by the heavy mechanical pump bolted to its main trunk. Up to this point, I participated voluntarily in this procedure. I could run for the hills at any time. Now, I'm connected to the IV tree. I'm in for the long haul. I'm not going anywhere.

June 8, Day -6

After a couple of hours of sleep in unfamiliar surroundings, a nurse woke me up ready to administer the first of 4 chemotherapy treatments. I learned my first lesson about hospital treatments. The preparation or the treatment would typically occur at the most inconvenient time possible. The hospital operated in full function mode 24 hours a day and didn't waste any of the overnight hours.

The second lesson was that a full night of sleep must be detrimental, and steps will be taken to wake a patient every hour or two no matter what.

The third lesson was that the preparation for the treatment took much longer than the treatment itself.

Those three lessons had no exceptions.

Preparation for the first of four heavy chemotherapy treatments began at 1:00 a.m. The treatment would start at 3:00 a.m. and continue until 8:00 a.m. Lab tests and vital signs would be evaluated regularly during the five-hour infusion process. So much for the idea of getting any sleep these first four nights of chemotherapy. The realization that the chemotherapy application was intended to kill all the cancerous stem cells in my body along with all of my bone marrow was enough to keep me awake anyway. What else would it kill or damage?

"It depends," the nurse said.

I've heard that before.

"Everyone has a different reaction. We'd have to wait and see."

I was sure that no patient ever reported growing more hair, getting healthier or becoming more attractive because of a heavy dose of chemotherapy.

The chemotherapy treatments were a combination of Busulfan, Fludarabine, and Cladribine. A patient education brochure described each drug, the reasons for use, and the long list of side effects that I didn't allow myself to read. The doctors and nurses described them well, and I knew it wasn't going to be a picnic. I knew this ride would be rough. I just didn't know how rough it would be.

I tried to nap a little after each of the four chemotherapy treatments. In the afternoon, Cindy and I walked the hallways of the 18th floor. The success of the stem cell transplantation process increases if patients can be kept in a sterile environment with an absence of germs, viruses or other unwelcome bacteria. Patients are encouraged to leave the room but were not allowed to leave the floor. There were too many germs on the other levels of the hospital or complex. Vacating the room required a surgical mask and a pair of latex gloves. So, I donned my gear and headed for the door along with my new friend, the IV tree, to which I was permanently attached and receiving fluids. I enjoyed getting out of the room and stretching my legs.

Like walking away from a bad accident, I felt remarkably good after that first treatment. I expected much worse and took advantage of my good fortune by walking the hallways at a pretty good clip. There were 48 other patients on this floor, and I met many of them while walking "laps" around the interior. Each lap was .2 miles so five laps would equal a mile. A mile was a piece of cake even wheeling around the IV tree with the mechanical pump and bags of fluid attached. An observant and bright-eyed assistant rewarded completed laps with a sticker that I would apply to my large hospital room door. You wanted the doctors to see a lot of stickers on your door, but you didn't want the other patients to think you were showing off or sucking up to the nurses.

Cindy has the blessing and the gift of casual conversation and a desire to meet new people. She accompanied me on each walking adventure, so we got to know our fellow patients quickly. Those relationships served as further incentive to get out of the room and walk the halls more often. We would look in the family lounge on our floor every time we passed it to see who was gathering. A wall of picture windows made the lounge a great place to meet, brew a cup of coffee, enjoy the downtown view and watch the sunsets.

Each of the next four days had a similar agenda. Five hours of chemotherapy, nap, eat, watch TV and walk the halls. Each day, however, the side effects became a lot more intense. I began to feel the delayed effects of that accident I thought I had walked away from. Headaches, nausea, and dizziness would interfere with the agenda along with trying to adapt to much less sleep and the monotonous routine. I built a sizable library of helicopter photos taken with my phone as they approached from every possible angle to drop off their patients. My family and friends are probably tired of receiving the pictures. I had plenty of time to text Jim on the 17th floor and took full advantage. He felt the same kind of side effects getting worse by the day.

Marc: Are you getting out and around any?

107

> **Jim:** Walked 3 times. I'm getting nauseated a lot. I'm trying not to complain but this isn't good.

> **Marc:** No. It sucks big time. My big issues are headaches, nausea and sleep deprivation. I have to get through one more night of chemo.

> **Jim:** Me, too. Headaches, nausea, shortness of breath.

After two days to rest, manage the chemotherapy side effects and flush the chemo drugs from my system, I was ready for the new cancer-free stem cells. I was jittery and nervous at this stage knowing the healthy stem cells had not yet been harvested. I was jumping off the high dive not knowing if the pool has been filled with water. You had to go with the promise that the water would reach the safe level a few seconds before you made the splash. There were a thousand things that could go wrong with the donor or the apheresis process, and my tired mind found a way to over analyze each one. What if he changed his mind? What if something came up? What if he got sick? Since my donor resided on another continent, there were another thousand variables that could prevent the fresh, healthy stem cells from arriving. The doctors had already destroyed my bone marrow and stem cells. What if there were no new cells to replace them? Those doctors assured me that everything was proceeding on schedule and that there was no need to worry. That helped. Not.

June 14, Day Zero

I had dreaded this day since I knew it was possible. I hoped I could avoid it, but deep down inside I knew transplant day would come. I was excited about it at the same time. While it wasn't easy, the stem cell transplant was the only road to recovery even if recovery was short-lived. The nurse on duty made the official announcement.

"We call this Day Zero," she said as she spelled it out with a marker on my white board. "Think of this as your second birthday."

I didn't buy that designation. That sounded too much like being born again which had happened many years before. Let's call it my third birthday.

"Each day after the transplant we'll add one with a plus sign," the nurse explained. "Tomorrow will be day +1. The day after will be +2."

Don't you think it's a little ironic? A man believes his days are numbered, and the transplant team begins to number his days. At least now the numbers are getting bigger.

The best gift I received on my third birthday was a big bag of life-giving stem cells. The donor had done the giving and, his healthy cells were on their way. I was humbled knowing that someone I had never met went out of his way and endured some considerable discomfort to donate the cells. I feel indebted to the medical team that flew these freshly harvested stem cells across the Atlantic Ocean directly to MD Anderson. I am grateful for the Houston team that analyzed and processed the cells upon arrival. It sure seemed like a lot of fuss for one old guy living in Houston with bone marrow cancer.

My anticipation and anxiety level is at least at Defcon 2. Chemotherapy had destroyed my bone marrow, stem cells and who knows what. There were still so many things to worry about that could crop up and sabotage the process.

The nurse on duty announced a schedule delay pushing back the transplant until noon. Take the anxiety level up a notch to Defcon 3. Jim was on the same schedule, and his stem cells had arrived. His donor was a 27-year-old male from the southern United

States. The cells had cleared the processing team, and the infusion was underway.

> **Jim: The nurse just walked in and set the time for transplant at 10:30 am. Premed at 10:00 am. 20 minutes to take off. Make sure all seats are in their upright position and all trays and tables stowed.**

> **Marc: Hey, you're at cruising altitude now! This is what we came here for, right? Know we are praying that all goes well. And, no puking!**

> **Jim: Amen, brother!**

Jim and I had made a bet after hearing that severe nausea would be one of the main side effects of chemo and the stem cell infusion. The first one to vomit had to pay the other $20.00.

My infusion was delayed again to later in the afternoon. Defcon 4. Then again to early evening. Now we're up to Defcon 5. My nerves were at their limits, and I was closing in on my very last one. Finally, the announcement came. The stem cells had arrived, and the infusion time rescheduled for 8:00 p.m. The leading stem cell doctor on duty would oversee the process accompanied by several nurses and physician assistants. Final preparations were underway, and my room was looking more like the lobby of this busy hotel.

Earlier in the afternoon, a nurse noticed the desktop cross, the framed scripture hanging on the wall and my Bible on the nightstand. He asked if I would like to have my stem cells blessed by a chaplain. I eagerly accepted that invitation, and the pastor of a local church stopped by about an hour before the transplant. We had a chance to talk and that supernatural peace began to settle over me

110

again. The chaplain looked at the posted scripture a few times but didn't ask why I had chosen that verse. I was ready to explain, but I guess it spoke for itself. As the transplant team arrived, each person took their place in the room. And, finally, the nurse walked in holding the coral colored plastic bag of several million stem cells and placed it on the IV tree. What a relief. I could finally exhale. The new cells were here and ready for transplant. I could see them, and I couldn't help thinking that this bag of cells could potentially help extend my life a few years. At least there was a 50/50 chance. Like McGyver attaching a homemade contraption that would avert disaster at the last second, a nurse connected the plastic tube extending from the stem cell bag to the CVC line in my chest.

The touching scene a few minutes before the stem cell release sticks in my memory and is one of the most vivid of the entire ordeal. Cindy and the transplant team stood with heads bowed and eyes closed.

"Dear Heavenly Father..." the Chaplain began the prayer as he asked God to bless these stem cells and to deliver their promise of healing and restoration. It was a beautiful scene, and I needed it. I had confidence in MD Anderson, the superior technology and the exceptional transplant team. But my faith and trust were in the Lord. The beautifully articulated blessing sealed the deal. I was ready. The nurse opened the valves, and the stem cells and a little extra measure of God-given peace began to flow down the tube and into my bloodstream.

Chapter 10
Post-Transplant

June 15, Day +1

A good night's sleep is like a snowstorm in south Texas. It's not impossible, but it doesn't come around often. I was more likely to see Texans' linebacker J.J. Watt walking through my oversized door in a pair of pink shoes than get a few hours of real sleep. Naps are the better description of the rest I'm getting and those occur with a little more frequency through the night and following day. As I woke up on the morning after absorbing a new set of stem cells and several of those welcome naps, I took an assessment of my physical and mental condition. I could feel the damaging effects of the four-day chemo cycle but nothing I could relate directly to the infusion of stem cells. I wasn't feeling any better, younger or more energetic. I had no urges to play soccer, no new appetite for European foods or any other new habits I could attribute to the donor. But I was still here, alive and awake.

The 18th-floor exercise class scheduled that day sounded like a good idea. It might even take my mind off the aches, pains and the constant sickness in my stomach. Other stem cell patients would be telling stories, and it was the only time patients from the 17th floor were allowed to visit the 18th floor. Jim might be there, and it would be one of the few opportunities to see how he was doing with a visual inspection. He sent a text message reply to my invitation telling me he wouldn't be able to attend.

113

Jim: I had a better night but my hgb is low. If I wasn't getting a transfusion of 2 units of blood right now you'd be seeing me. Have a good time.

Marc: Just wasn't the same without you. It was good to get out of the room, though. We're getting a new crop of patients in the classes. Several were in the chemo stage.

Jim: Yeah, we're next on that list. I started early. Blood levels crash and incontinence sets in. It's something to look for the end of.

I wasn't sure what Jim meant by being next on the list. We'd already had our four days of chemo before the stem cell infusion. Then, out of left field comes another gut punch. More chemo. The nurse came in with a new set of fluid bags and announced there would be two more days of chemotherapy. Jim's text message warned of another unexpected round of chemo packing a crushing right hook. This chemo was intended to prevent the new stem cells from attacking my healthy tissues and organs. I was fully aware that prevention drugs would be needed, but I didn't anticipate that it would be more chemotherapy. And, this chemo cycle would finish the job that the first cycle started.

This chemo cycle and an adverse reaction to the stem cells would take me and my new friend Jim down for the count.

Jim: Tacrolimus is my GVHD drug. Causes headaches. I'm sure they will fill you in on the fun stuff. I've had the 2 bags of blood then Tacro for 2 days. Antibiotics for precaution.

> **Marc: I'm getting more chemo tomorrow for GVHD. A drug called Cytoxan. It beats up the bladder, so they will triple my fluid levels beginning at 4:00 am. The strategy for the day is 'drink and pee.' The 2 hours of chemo starts at 9:00 am.**

The roughest time is the first few days after the stem cell transplant, and all eyes are on me. How sick will he get? What problems will develop? Will his body reject the new stem cells? Will those new cells start attacking healthy tissues? I felt like a lab rat injected with a new test substance. Something was going to happen, but no one could anticipate what that would be.

June 17, Day +3

Four things are wreaking havoc on this aching body of mine. It's still reeling from the first round of chemo. It's trying to rally from the two additional chemotherapy blasts. This body is fighting the foreign stem cells. And, it's absorbing new anti-rejection drugs. I'm spending most of my time in bed hoping to get through the next 24 hours. I would soon reach the pit. The low point of the transplant. I couldn't help but think about the 20% to 30% of patients who don't survive the transplant process. I was sure this phase claimed many of them.

It's hard to think about anything other than how bad you feel on the way to the pit. Whenever I could set those thoughts aside, I spent the time lying awake in prayer and meditation. The knowledge that God was in control was more than comforting. The knowledge that He knew exactly where I was and what I was going through gave me supernatural confidence and the determination to fight through this phase. In the early morning hours, I asked God to direct me and guide my steps according to His promises in the Word. Then I started thinking of all the things I couldn't do. I was stuck in a hospital. I could barely move. My contacts were limited. I was in a lot of pain. I was telling God I was available for His service but with a long list of conditions. I couldn't even finish the thought before I received a convicting response. *What's with all the conditions? Why are you presenting all these excuses? Don't you know who you are talking to? I provide the strength, the power, and the ability to do anything I ask you to do. Stop with the excuses, already!* The powerful conviction hit me square in the heart, but it was gladly received and well deserved. I smiled a massive ear to ear smile, thanked the Holy Spirit for the correction and dozed off for one of those rare short naps feeling secure in the palm of God's hand.

I hardly noticed it was Father's Day until I got another text from Jim.

Jim: Happy Father's Day! I hope you are doing well today. One more bag of blood makes a total of seven so far.

> **Marc: Happy Father's Day back at 'cha. I've had a rough couple of days. This new chemo is kicking my butt. I owe you $20.00. I puked last night.**

> **Jim: Yeah, and I'll give it right back. I wish I had lost several times. This is day +4 and I have lots of diarrhea. I'm holding fluids, too. I now weigh 5 pounds more than at check in.**

> **Marc: I have a bad case of the scoots myself. I ate breakfast yesterday but not much since. The heavy fluids will end at 2:00 pm for me.**

> **Jim: They are trying to slow me down with Imodium.**

Texting with Jim helps take my mind off of all my physical problems and think about someone else's health issues. The people around me focus entirely on how I feel and how I'm reacting. I appreciate the attention, but when everyone's focus is exclusively on you, and you're fighting some debilitating side effects, it takes some effort to think about something else. Texting is a welcome diversion.

June 20, Day +6

A new patient moved into the room next to mine on the 18th floor. Jacob came prepared for the 30-day ordeal. He brought blank canvases to paint, wooden models to assemble and other activities to keep him busy for months. I couldn't even imagine trying to paint, assemble anything or expect the tiniest spark of creativity. His optimism was contagious, and he walked the halls with a pre-transplant briskness full of nervous energy. He dialed back his pace and allowed me to join him for a few steps knowing it took every ounce of effort I had. In one of our hallway conversations, he confided that his stem cell transplant was his best and last hope. He would be in serious trouble if the transplant didn't work. Jacob suffered from Multiple Myeloma, a form of cancer that attacks the plasma cells and wreaks havoc on red blood cells, bones, and kidneys. Jacob was a week or so behind me in the transplant process, but since he was receiving his own stem cells, the process would move a little faster for him.

There was a mix of transplant types on the 18th floor. Some patients like me received stem cells from a related or unrelated donor. Those are called allogenic stem cell transplants. Another group of patients received their own stem cells harvested a few weeks before the transplant. Those are called autologous transplants. The stem cells are collected from the patient and frozen before transplant conditioning. Their stem cells are healthy but would be damaged or destroyed by chemotherapy. After the treatments, they are infused with their stem cells to resume the process of producing healthy red and white blood cells and platelets. Autologous stem cell transplant patients endure a difficult treatment process but recover faster from the transplant since their body doesn't reject the stem cells.

When the frozen stem cells are prepared and infused into an autologous transplant patient, it produces a nasty and pervasive odor for a day or two like a pan of creamed corn burned on the stove. It permeates their room and the airspace about six feet around them. The nurses were used to the toxic smell, but Cindy and I had to hold our noses when walking by one of their rooms. We would keep a polite distance from them if they were out and about. The patient becomes desensitized and can't smell it after a while but everyone else can. They can't smell it but the patient can see the odor in the facial expressions and reactions of everyone around them. We had to stay away from Jacob for a couple of days.

The next 48 hours were agonizing. Blood counts are crashing, and the chemo side effects were worsening. The chemotherapy wreaks havoc on the body's gastrointestinal system. One of the nurses said that it damages everything from the mouth to the rear end and I'm feeling every part of it. Jim is too, and I haven't heard from him in a few days.

Jim: My mouth pain is so severe it hurts to text. I've been out of it for a while. We will make it through this. You still with me up there?

Marc: I'm still with you. Hanging on by my fingernails. I can't come up with a body part that doesn't hurt. OxyContin is helping the headaches. Zofran is keeping me from barfing. But we will get through this. Irritation #1: The Tacrolimus pump on

> the tree. This thing starts beeping every 90 minutes or so around the clock. Is yours doing that?

> **Marc:** By the way, I'm eating presoaked mushy Raisin Bran sans raisins. Not bad and you can swallow it if you let it soak long enough.

> **Jim:** Texting has become very difficult for me. My pump beeps every three minutes.

Both Jim and I are now in the midst of the most difficult physical challenge of our lives. My white blood cell count has completely flatlined. The reading has been 0.0 for the past couple of days. I can hardly raise my head. Everything hurts except my stomach which is continuously on the verge of hurling its contents. I feel like I've been hit by a truck right after running two marathons. Bowel movements are excruciating. Getting to the bathroom is a significant challenge. Even the sunlight coming in through the small window is extremely painful. Cindy sees me wince from the light, so she lowers the window shade a little more to help block the painful contrast. My perspective was changing from day to day to hour by hour. You pray for the strength to endure a little more pain and get through the next hour.

Like the dessert cart at a nice restaurant, nurses offer four pain relievers on a type of opiate menu rolled in for circumstances like these. The first pain relief option I tried was Tramadol, which is like fresh fruit with a dab of whipped cream. It was sweet but still had some nutritional value. Tramadol worked well for a day or so. The next option, OxyContin, has a little more sugar in it. I've heard so many bad things about OxyContin that I'm deathly afraid of getting anywhere near it. If your pain is unbearable, you can take another step up and try Dilaudid. Since one of the major side effects

119

of Dilaudid is headaches, it didn't seem to make much sense. The most sugar on the dessert cart is in morphine, and I want no part of it. However, my splitting headaches are so severe that I'm willing to try something that I would otherwise never consider.

Instead of a one-time dessert, I asked the nurses for a pain relief plan that I could regularly take to maintain some level of the drug in my system. If I could take the edge off the pain, perhaps it would be more manageable. The nurses would not comply with that request stating that I was to decide how much pain relief I needed and when to take it. Did I need a little taste of sugar or a big piece of chocolate cake? They were serving drugs to treat the pain I had at that moment and wouldn't hear of an ongoing plan. They did an excellent job of informing me of the options but stopped short of a professional recommendation which I found odd and incredibly frustrating. I was expected to make an informed medical decision at the lowest, most painful point in my recovery. I regret the tone of voice I used to express how annoyed I was.

The doctors and nurses were adamant about patients describing their symptoms in as much detail as possible. A good doctor needs detailed information to treat a patient properly. I get that. But if I expressed my pain, they would prescribe pain relief depending on where I placed that pain on a scale of 1 to 10. If I reported nausea, there would be a medication prescribed for that. Playing the tough guy or enduring the symptoms was discouraged in favor of addressing the symptoms directly. I felt a lot of pressure to describe every symptom and take every medication prescribed to weather the tough days with as much comfort as possible. I appreciated their approach and their good intentions, but sometimes the treatment and its side effects seem worse than the symptoms.

Thinking back to the monthly chemotherapy treatments before the transplant, splitting headaches along with nausea, dizziness, weakness, and fatigue were common side effects. God tested me back then when the headache pain was the most intense with a promise to relieve that pain. I was to endure the other symptoms but trust Him with the headache pain. He had tested me in different ways before and even though I hadn't passed every test, I had learned to trust him. Once again, He was true to His word. What headaches I had were minimal and easy to bear. The other symptoms like fatigue and nausea were challenging but manageable.

During the most painful headaches I had after the transplant, God spoke to me again. Through my ear-splitting headaches crushing the back of my head, He reminded me of His grace and how He had relieved the headaches caused by the earlier chemotherapy treatments. In the midst of my greatest discomfort, I hadn't even thought of appealing to my Father for relief. He convicted me of that oversight and commanded that I trust Him for relief. I said I'd trust Him with the headaches, but I was no match for the pressure applied by the doctors and nurses. They wouldn't buy anything close to a statement that I had no headaches and required no pain relief. When that sense of peace came over me again, I believed He would handle that as well.

The pain continued to intensify, and I was close to my breaking point. It was decision time. Do I take a pain reliever or trust God to take away the pain? I confess to a moment of doubt, but I knew deep down that my faith and trust would be rewarded. It always was.

The life of a believer isn't a spectator sport. It requires active participation. Things don't just happen. God is always working behind the scenes, but He doesn't snap his fingers and relieve pain. A step of faith is required. The believer spends time in prayer. They demonstrate humility. They make a specific request with the belief that an answer will be forthcoming. God sees that faith, extends his hand and offers his grace. That offer must be accepted. God must be trusted. The issue must be fully submitted to God. God's commands must be obeyed. Finally, faith gets the action going. My moment was at hand requiring deep faith and action on my part.

What would you do? Trust in modern medicine to relieve the excruciating pain or take a leap of faith and give the headaches to God? Did I hear God correctly or was I delusional and imagining the whole thing?

God reminded me that He was much bigger than the most painful headache I could imagine. And, much bigger than any medicine that was in current use or would ever be invented. I decided to go all in and give the headaches to God.

Good call. It should be no surprise that the pain subsided the next day. I had a host of other issues but the headaches, the worst and most painful of them all, were gone. And, so was the pressure from the nurses. The nurses didn't bring up the subject, and neither did I. The stem cell doctor making the rounds didn't even ask about the headaches during her daily visit. I didn't complain about headache pain, and the nurses didn't prescribe any more pain relievers. The headache pain relief made the other symptoms more manageable and provided a welcome reminder that God was in control, knew exactly what was going on and was with me in that hospital room. What a difference. Maybe, just maybe I could survive this ordeal.

With spiritual assurance, a loving wife who wouldn't leave my side and an incredible medical team, I felt like I could weather any storm. And, this one was a monster. It could curl my hair if I had any.

More and more of my short grey hairs were showing up on my clothing and pillowcase than on my head. It started with a few here and a few there, but now the hair fell out in clumps. Arms, legs, underarms. No hair on my body was safe. I helped it along with a tug or two, but it wasn't long before I had a shiny bald head. The intense chemotherapy before the transplant had taken its toll.

Usually, this kind of transformation would have been emotionally devastating. Compared to everything else I had going on, the hair loss seemed to be the least of my worries. Plus, all my new friends shared the same hairstyle, and the bald head was considered a badge of honor. It's one more thing requiring some adaptation.

June 26, Day +12

I've lost track, but the whiteboard near the hospital room door says it's day +12 and I'm hoping to bottom out soon. Would there be a moment when I felt any better? Would this downward spiral of hurting more, feeling sicker or losing ground ever end? I feel awful in so many ways and need to touch base with Jim.

> **Marc: Hey, buddy! This is day 6 with a 0.0 white blood cell count. I get 2 units of blood today and I've gained 10 lbs in fluid weight. Everything hurts and I'm pretty much spent. Other than that, I feel pretty good. My body hair started coming out in clumps a couple of days ago. Darn hair is getting all over everything. These are the rough days. You must feel bad, too. But we'll get through it. One day at a time.**

> **Jim: Together is the word. I'll be getting blood this afternoon again for the low Hgb. We are on track from what they tell me. It's a process. I have great nurses and attendants. We'll have to have a party when we leave. I'm losing my hair, too. Chest hair doesn't have a home anymore. Arm hair hanging in.**

> **Jim: I have lesions top to bottom. Even on my scrotum. The ones in my mouth are actually getting better.**

123

> **Marc:** Not scrotum lesions! I have those, too! What are you putting on yours? I'm trying aloe vera gel but I can't recommend it yet. I have lesions in my armpits, also.

> **Marc:** Damn scrotum lesions!

> **Jim:** Gold Bond Original Powder. I'm going dry and commando. And, yes, I can recommend it. It works. I'll catch up with you soon. These lesions have got to go.

A strong support group is helpful if you have to go through a health crisis like this. While Cindy and the nursing team are exceptional, knowing your experiences are not unique and being able to communicate with another patient is reassuring. Jim has been the friend I needed and the teammate I had anticipated.

After seven days of the worst physical anguish I have ever experienced, I needed to hear some good news. I needed a turning point. I was reaching and needed to grab something tangible. After being in the bottom of this pit so long, I needed a lifeline. It came with the daily blood test results. A few brave white blood cells had decided to make a home in my bloodstream. My white blood cell count had rocketed up from 0.0 to a 0.2 reading. Could there be more tomorrow? Could I inch a little closer to the normal range of 4.5 to 11.0?

> **Jim:** How are your numbers today? I still have some lesions, too. The one in my throat is really painful. It takes me forever to swallow my pills.

> **Marc:** I jumped up to a .2 WBC today. Hallelujah! After 7 days at 0.0, it's nice to see a small step in the right direction. Platelets are at 33. Hgb is 9.2. So, no blood or platelet

transfusions today. Swelling is my big issue now. Legs and ankles are big and tight. I've had Lasix for the past 2 days. I hate the Lasix. I spend half the day in the bathroom negotiating with my bowels and urinary tract. I won't even talk about the lesions in my nether regions. I also have a weird bacteria in my blood. They are working on a specific antibiotic to address it. It seems to be responding to the general antibiotic they are using now.

A platelet count below 10 causes extreme fatigue, weakness, and dizziness and usually triggers an infusion. Receiving platelets is like any other infusion except the fluid is a golden-brown color and the process involves a few extra steps. A dose of industrial strength Benadryl would decrease allergic reactions like hives and itching. Regular blood tests would expose any other physical response that would require immediate attention.

One of those blood tests revealed an unusual bacteria. The nurse made a call and before you could say "bone marrow biopsy," lab technicians in white coats filled the room doing further tests on my blood. I couldn't see much, but I could hear the clanking of glass containers and the shuffling activity of the technicians. Their muffled conversations carried some urgency and concern. The lab team identified the bacteria as "Capnocytophaga Sputigena," and testing began to replicate the bacteria in the lab, monitor its growth and develop an antibiotic that would effectively attack it. I took what the doctors called a broad spectrum antibiotic while waiting for the custom version.

Just when you think you have seen every skill and discipline, here come the lab technicians and the infectious disease specialists. Their speed and ability to identify the bacteria quickly was beyond impressive. I was continually blown away by the depth and range of the medical expertise at MD Anderson. It seems no matter what happened there was a team of experts ready to address that specific issue at that exact moment. I was impressed and humbled every day and thankful to be there. I couldn't help but be thankful that all this time, all this effort, and all this experience was focused on getting me through this ordeal and on to a few more healthy years on this planet. It's good to know we live in a world where the goodness and compassion of others are clearly on display.

There are two distinctly different worlds. There is the world we see on the news where everyone is angry and divided. The other is the one right in front of you with love, kindness, and goodwill all around. Being able to see that contrast with full clarity is another benefit of going through a trial like this. I'll take the latter view, thank you.

It was time for a bold decision and declaration. Stem cell transplant survivors often talk about their worst day with an element of pride. They are happy to have survived and not bashful in describing the worst day of the ordeal. Ben from Kansas City named day +3 as his worst day during a recent hallway conversation. He endured his transplant a couple of weeks ago. He looked back on the pain and lack of any continence and was relieved that those days were behind him. I needed to make a similar declaration. The last day with the 0.0 white blood cell count would be the worst day of this experience. The low point. I would just make it so. Every day going forward would be better than that day. The sign of a few fearless white blood cells showing up in my lab tests would signal better days ahead. I had to get out of bed, eat what I could, take a few steps, and then plow through a few more no matter how painful or difficult. Cindy was in full support mode and provided that helping hand to guide me through that process and encourage me to continue down this new path.

Chapter 11

Early Recovery

June 27, Day +13

The worst day of the stem cell transplant ordeal was indeed day +13, the last of the seven days with the 0.0 white blood cell count. Fortunately, a rope ladder extended to the bottom of that painful pit with Cindy on the other end encouraging me to climb up. One painful step at a time, a little improvement came my way with each following day. I spent more and more time out of bed able to walk the halls, gain some strength and eat a little. The days of big meals were long gone. My sick stomach couldn't handle much food at one time. Small meals sprinkled throughout the day would have to sustain me now and for months to come.

Each day the walks got a little easier. I got out of bed a little faster and added another bite or two to each meal. While running a marathon was out of the question, day 30 in the hospital was approaching, and I was looking forward to a change of scenery.

The daily labs continued, and my white blood cell count continued to rise. The doctors were looking for a white blood cell count of 2.0 before they would consider a release from the hospital in addition to an absolute neutrophil reading of 1.5. That became my target, as if there was anything I could do to influence those numbers. The other criteria for release included a reduction in side effects, medications had to be taken by mouth, no fevers could be present, and I had to be capable of drinking two liters of water per day. Once I passed those tests, I would be a free man. One more hurdle remained. I had to shake that pesky bacteria.

The bacteria would not let go and proved to be the biggest obstacle to my release. I saw the infectious disease team every day and despite the best efforts of the lab technicians, the custom antibiotic they were looking for eluded them. An intelligent looking young doctor conveyed the bad news.

"It's going to take another ten days to get rid of the bacteria," the doctor said. "We'll get it out of your system with the broad-spectrum antibiotic. It's just going to take a little longer than we expected."

I tried to duck, but the punch landed squarely on my gut. Another week and a half? How could I do that? Even though I met the other release criteria, the doctors suggested I stay in the hospital until it they could confirm that the bacteria was gone.

Like many other things, the final decision fell to me. I could demand a release and take my chances or play it safe in the hospital until the blood tests showed no signs of the bacteria.

What would you do?

It was tempting to seize the moment and run for the hills. I had been in the hospital for four weeks and was ready to limp, skip, crawl, whatever I had to do to get out the front door. The doctors wouldn't release me under any circumstances where I would be in any real danger, right? Jim on the 17th floor was going to be released soon, and he couldn't leave without me. I couldn't let that happen, could I?

That sense of peace swept over me again, and I told the stem cell doctor we had come too far and been through too much to leave now without a clean bill of health. He had worked too hard. The nurses had put in too much effort. The lab technicians had devoted too much time for me to roll the dice and put all that effort at risk.

We would stay and let them finish their work. We wanted to be an absolute success story they could celebrate, and we had no desire to return to this or any other hospital.

July 2, Day +18

Two days later the doctor conveyed another piece of good news. The infectious disease team had identified another antibiotic that was more sensitive to the bacteria we were fighting. They were 95% certain this antibiotic would finish off the bacteria and could confidently release me from the confines of the 18th floor. We grabbed that opportunity and prepared for our release. It took all of 10 minutes to gather up our belongings and the gifts and trinkets we had acquired over the last 30 days.

The release process would take a little longer. There were doctors to see, forms to fill out and final tests to take. And, there was the issue of that bacteria. The infectious disease doctors suspected that the CVC port in my chest may be harboring some of the remaining bacteria and wanted to remove it before my release. A specialist in port removal came up to my room and started the procedure right then and there. She must have walked right off the Seinfeld set talking Cindy and me through the preparation steps with a few one-liners and hospital jokes.

"Grab the rail and take a deep breath," she warned.

With a skillful tug at precisely the right time, the specialist removed the CVC port with no anesthesia and relatively little pain. My worry and anxiety over the removal process proved to be unfounded. She continued her light-hearted routine as she patched up the hole in my chest. I don't know which felt better, the port removal or the belly laughs.

My chest and right arm needed a few days to heal before they could insert a new line. That meant three free days to sleep, shower and move about with no tubes attached and no IV tree following me around. Like a dog on a short leash, I felt like I'd been unhooked and turned loose to run around the backyard for a couple of days. It's only 72 hours, but I'll take it.

The hospital leash was a little longer but still present. I could leave the campus, but I had to stay close to MD Anderson's emergency room. I couldn't venture further than 15 minutes away for the next 60 days. If I picked up a graft-versus-host disease, infection, bleeding, had an emergency relapse or a new problem or issue developed, it would most likely occur in that 60-day period. It took a good hour to drive home on a good day and traffic could delay the commute another hour. That was too risky, so we moved to a nearby furnished apartment for a two or three-month stay.

We also got a good lecture and a list of "Do's and Don'ts" from a survivorship nurse named Karen before we could go. The "Do's" were few. Do submit to the watchful eye of a "round the clock" caregiver. Wear a surgical mask anytime I was likely to be in a crowd or group of people. Drink two liters of water a day and walk as much as I could. Wash my filthy hands, the entry point for most diseases and bacteria, frequently.

The "Don'ts" were many and avoiding people and crowds topped the long list. Don't go around sick people, gyms, zoos, and pools. Sadly, churches were also on the taboo list. With all the handshaking, hugging and contact with large groups of people, I could understand why attending a church service could be a problem. I'd have to find a creative solution to that one. Don't let any visitors with coughs or sore throats into our apartment. Don't eat any fresh fruits or vegetables. Those are prohibited. Food ordered at a restaurant had to be cooked to order and cooked thoroughly. Don't eat at a buffet. Any foods that had been sitting around in a salad bar or a soup bowl were strictly off limits. Finally,

I was to stay away from plants, pets, and children under 12. Those kids are germ magnets!

I'll spare you the list of conditions which would require a return to the emergency room. These were common symptoms of graft-versus-host disease (GVHD) that would concentrate in the skin, stomach or liver. Cindy would watch for those. The Do's and Don'ts nurse made it painfully clear. I had no immune system, and no matter what I wanted to believe, I wasn't well yet. I could leave the hospital but had to be careful where I went and what I did. My body couldn't fight even the most common everyday germs. Dr. Kornblau had the best advice.

"Treat him like a newborn baby," he said. "Not the second or third child, though. Over protect him like you do your first child."

Short-term housing is in high demand in the Medical Center, and there are numerous options near MD Anderson. We decided on a furnished apartment across the street from Hermann Park a mile north of MD Anderson and a five-minute drive to the parking garage. Hermann Park is a beautiful open 445-acre green space in the heart of Houston. It was donated to the City of Houston in 1914 and encompasses a golf course, the Houston Zoo, Miller Outdoor Theater, the eight-acre McGovern Lake, Japanese Gardens and the Herman Park Railroad offering a 20-minute train ride around and through the park. The train ride and the hungry ducks at McGovern Lake were favorites of my oldest grandchild during visits in younger and healthier days. The park attracts over six million visitors each year.

A monument depicting Sam Houston on horseback watches over the park atop a 35-foot marble pedestal. Sam Houston has pointed visitors towards the park and the San Jacinto Monument several miles away since 1925 and is a reminder of the city's storied history.

The apartment was an easy walk to the Marvin Taylor Trail, a two-mile exercise trail around the golf course. It's a beautiful walk around the green spaces, ponds and lush landscaping with moss-covered oak trees lining the gravel trail. I had high hopes of mastering this trail and using it to restore my running legs during my two-month stay. Weaker than expected muscles and the oppressive summer heat and humidity would complicate that plan.

The apartment was also a short drive to Houston's Museum District, an internationally recognized art center. Walkers can visit most of the 19 museums that make up the Museum District on foot along tree-lined streets, established neighborhoods and a few more of those moss-draped oak trees. The Museum District is home to the Museum of Fine Arts, Houston, the sixth largest art museum in the nation, founded in 1900. The Museum of Natural Science is also a favorite along with the Contemporary Art Museum and others covering a broad cultural spectrum. We have lived in Houston for over 15 years and only visited a few of these great museums. We set a goal to visit every one of them over the next two months.

Wasting time moping around an apartment seemed like such a bad idea compared with all the things to do such a short distance away. That was the clear-headed thinking of a few months ago. Those world-class attractions would serve as motivation to get outside and accomplish something positive during my 60-day restriction period.

July 3, Day +19

The day of my release finally came. After 27 days on the 18th floor, we packed our acquired belongings and a shopping bag full of prescriptions into a car covered with a month's worth of dirt. We paid an exorbitant parking fee and drove to a nearby hotel. I wanted to shout in my best Braveheart William Wallace voice,

132

"Freedom!" No IV trees, no tubes, no nurses and no chores like measuring personal waste. I felt like I was experiencing an incredible new world. The bright sunlight on a warm July afternoon made me squint and reach for the sunglasses in the car right where I had left them four weeks ago.

I reserved our furnished apartment before being admitted to the hospital but missed the move in date by two days. Not to let an opportunity pass us by, Cindy and I treated ourselves to a fancy hotel suite and turned those days into a mini vacation. The small one-bedroom suite felt like the Royal Plaza Suite overlooking Manhattan at the Plaza Hotel. The first night was a slice of heaven, and we felt like royals. The opportunity to sleep in a luxurious king size bed with no noise and interruptions was undoubtedly a royal treatment. I still woke up frequently for runs to the restroom but what an improvement. The morning shower was another blessing. It was a real shower that felt like a Hawaiian waterfall cascading down a mountain. I enjoyed every luscious moment splashing about with no need for dodging around plastic tubes or IV trees. I forgot about feeling sick, tired and weak for the few brief moments of this little holiday. Never mind the fact that I felt so grateful to be alive, intact and out of a hospital room.

Daily visits to MD Anderson were required and didn't seem to be too much of an imposition. A large section of the 10th floor is reserved for infusions and follow up treatments for stem cell transplant patients. I shook hands with a new post-transplant team including a nurse, assistant, and pharmacist. They would monitor all the prescribed medications, examine me each day, review the lab work, and supervise infusions of fluids and other medications best administered by IV. Compared to the daily regimen in the hospital room, the three to four-hour visits were a piece of cake.

I was always instructed to wear a surgical mask at M D Anderson. There were a lot of people there with a wide range of ailments, viruses, bacteria, and germs and my immune system wasn't up to the task of fighting them off. I could catch anything. So now, I looked exactly like the cancer patients I viewed and felt badly for a few short months ago. Bald head? Check. Surgical mask? Check. Droopy shoulders? Check. Slower pace? Check. But, I also inherited some of their exceptional resilience. Fighting spirit? Check. Determination? Check. And, I was cold all the time. The temperature, no matter what the thermometer indicated, seemed to be a few degrees below my comfort level. Even in the hot summer months, many recovering cancer patients like me would sport warm-up suits and thick jackets that were so out of place for the season.

July 6, Day +22

As if recaptured by the English army, my three days of freedom were over. The leash free tail wagging ended with the installation of my new IV line. Since I had been through the most intense treatments, I was fortunate to receive a new PICC line (Peripherally Inserted Central Catheter) with two lumens instead of the CVC line with three lumens. You'll have to take my word for it. It makes a big difference.

The proper place for a PICC line is the right arm a few inches above the elbow. A skilled nurse, about an hour of time and a lot of lidocaine injections were required to complete the installation.

Here I am again, flat on my back looking up at some harsh hospital ceiling lights. Like the CVC line, the tube was skillfully inserted through the skin and directly into a large vein. The PICC line specialist guided a catheter into the main vein near the heart where the blood flows quickly. A little plastic hub keeps the tube in place attached to the skin by three stitches. Two lumens extend from the hub and serve as the connection for the IV fluids. A precautionary chest X-ray helps make sure all the tubes found their way to the right places and verify the success of the installation.

The PICC line would make the frequent infusions go much faster. Adapting to this new apparatus is no picnic but it's much less offensive than the CVC line. After a couple of weeks, you hardly know it's there.

I stayed on the recovery track with relatively few complications, and the hospital visits became less frequent. After a week of the daily hospital visits, the post-transplant team allowed me to infuse the fluids and magnesium I needed at home. Since I had the PICC line, the process would simple. The infuser is about the size of a softball connected to one end of a plastic tube. We would connect the other end to the purple lumen in my PICC line. It took about five hours to complete the infusion, but I could carry the infuser where ever I wanted to go. The nurses walked us through the process, and we confidently left the hospital with two of these premixed softball-size infusers that would get us through the weekend. Two days off! Hallelujah!

The recovery track, however, was a tough road. I felt sick most of the time and could never predict what the next day would bring. I had to fight through nausea, fatigue, dizziness, and weakness to get up and do the things I was now free to do and enjoy all those nearby attractions. I couldn't get enough sleep, and I was losing weight. Chemotherapy wiped out most of my taste buds and any semblance of an appetite. No foods had any appeal whatsoever. If Cindy hadn't been so insistent, I wouldn't have eaten anything at all. Jim had similar problems.

> **Jim: How did your day go? Mine wasn't so good.**

> **Marc: Mine was okay but not that great. I feel worn out and beat up. What's going on with you?**

135

Jim: Same. Fatigue nonstop. We're waiting for the shuttle. I'm walking around like I've got dropsy. Every time I see a chair my butt drops into it. There are times I wonder if I'm going to make it. I'm pretty strong, though. Tomorrow is another day. Better, I hope.

Marc: At least you're out and about. We ran a few errands today but that's about it. No doubt both of us will get through this thing but it's tough getting through each day. It will be nice once we get some energy back. Until then we just have to knock out one day at a time.

Jim: They stopped my energy vitamin about 3 weeks ago. I'm going to ask to add it back. The energy vitamin really helped before all this started. Unless it reacts with something else, they should allow it. I'll let you know.

A couple of days later I got a text from Jim at 4:00 in the morning.

Jim: I'm so close to going to the hospital. Are you up?

Marc: Just made another bathroom run. What is wrong?

Jim: Stomach mainly. I have taken antacids, nausea meds, pain pills. Can't sleep. Any suggestions?

Marc: I sleep sitting up when that happens. Or, try to. When I lie flat, everything starts to back up. When all else fails I drink a Diet Coke.

> **Jim:** I'll try the Diet Coke. Keep you posted.

> **Marc:** Usually, I take a Pepcid at bedtime and eat a few Tums every time I go to the bathroom. I sleep with my head elevated. It helps most of the time.

> **Jim:** I sure don't want to go back to the hospital. They might keep me.

> **Marc:** Make sure its Coke or Diet Coke.

> **Jim:** DC this time.

> **Marc:** Cool. A good burp or 2 will help.

July 14, Day +30

It's time for another look at my bone marrow to see if the transplant worked. A good biopsy report would show a low percentage of blasts or immature stem cells. The bone marrow should be denser, and there should be no trace of Myelodysplastic Syndrome. Lab results will also reveal the percentage of donor cells in the marrow. The best outcome would be 100%. My mutant cells out. Healthy donor cells in.

I've endured eight bone marrow biopsies to date but this one has me on edge. A good result means the stem cell transplant is working. A bad result could indicate that the MDS resisted the transplant and we'd be back to the drawing board with nothing to show for all the pain and suffering. The biopsy nurse completed the procedure without much fanfare. I would limp around for a couple of days then wait a few more days to get the results. The test would be the main topic of our next doctor visit and evaluation.

It was a rough week waiting for the bone marrow biopsy results. I couldn't stop thinking about how I might react. Would I shout for joy if the results were good? Could I battle back from the despondent feeling if the results were bad? I had plenty of other problems to think about during that week. There were long days at MD Anderson getting lab work and infusions. My platelets crashed requiring an additional infusion that caused an intense allergic reaction. Both lumens in my PICC line were blocked requiring a visit to the Infusion Therapy center. You didn't want to be sentenced to Infusion Therapy. Lines were long, and the wait could be a couple hours or more. Nausea became more extreme causing more bouts with vomiting. That on top of the usual weakness and nausea that was causing me so much grief.

July 19, Day +35

After one of the longest weeks of my life, the waiting was over. Cindy and I made our way to the Stem Cell Center on the 8th floor at MD Anderson and our appointment with Dr. Kornblau. Typically, these visits were routine and mostly uneventful, but this one was different. This was the big reveal. Did the transplant work? Did I have other problems and an even tougher road ahead? Had I run out of options?

We took our seats in the exam room and waited for Dr. Kornblau. After his signature knock, he opened the door, and I tried to read his face as he walked in and shook my hand. He skipped the small talk and went right to the news.

"Your bone marrow looks good," he said with a doctor-like poker face. The corners of his mouth turned up and he stopped trying to constrain his smile. "Looks like we got it."

I wanted to jump up and hug the doctor, but the man code and proper hospital protocol prohibited that kind of public display. A flow of tears streamed down Cindy's cheeks. The bone marrow biopsy results were better than good. They were better than we could have ever expected. The blast count was at 2% which is well within the normal range. Bone marrow cellularity was 40% which is twice the density that it was before the transplant. Donor cells were at or close to 100%. And finally, there was no trace of MDS in the marrow sample. None! I was officially in remission and cancer free. Cancer free! In the early stages of recovery, there is a 40% chance that the MDS could return. But for today, I'm in remission. Today, I'm cancer free!

I waved at the crowd as I rounded the bases after a grand slam home run to win the World Series. I spiked the football in the end zone after scoring a touchdown in overtime to win the Vince Lombardi Trophy and the Super Bowl. I raised my fist speeding past the checkered flag at the Indianapolis 500. At least it felt that way. The transplant was working. I was on the road to recovery and moving forward. That knowledge was a needed boost to get through the days and nights of discomfort and other challenges that awaited us. It was a quantum leap forward.

I had survived the most intense part of the transplant. The new stem cells found their rightful place. The old cancerous stem cells were dead and gone. The resistance my body was putting up to the new stem cells was manageable. I was on track and maybe a little ahead at this stage of the game. God had seen me through the darkest days, lifted me out of the pit, placed my feet on more solid ground, and now He was leading me through the recovery. That word sounds so sweet. Recovery.

Jim was out of the hospital as well. He and his lovely wife, Coleen, were staying in a nearby hotel with shuttle service to grocery stores, shopping centers, and medical facilities. Since we had a car, we could pick them up, see some sights and push the boundaries a little. It was always nice to see them; share our experiences and laugh at the contradictions and absurdities we had witnessed along the pathways of this journey. As much as Jim and I had to share, Cindy and Coleen had even more in common trying to provide caregiving services to cranky husbands who weren't always cooperative. They were in uncharted territory facing challenges they had never encountered before. They were seeing sides of their mates they had never seen before.

Jim battled many graft-versus-host diseases in the form of rashes, extreme nausea, diarrhea and stomach problems. The intense chemo ravaged his gastrointestinal tract. He was in and out of the hospital a time or two in addition to a couple of trips to the emergency room.

After getting the green light, some friends started to check in on us and our Medical Center living quarters. The fact that they would go out of their way to visit was comforting and encouraging. It was a welcome relief from the daily grind of pushing through all the discomforts to hear about their challenges and triumphs. They didn't have to bring anything or say anything in particular. Their presence was enough to provide a much-needed lift. My old bosses who had become good friends dropped by a couple of times. They filled me in on the latest gossip and big events at the former workplace and the updates served as a pleasant diversion. A couple of friends from church took me to lunch and brought me up to date on The Woodlands and the weekly discussion topics of our men's group. That group moved one of their meetings to the clubhouse at my temporary apartment home. It was a long drive for them and a major inconvenience. But, what a lift! Being included in the group once again deeply touched my heart and proved a tremendous boost to my spirits. I took no offense from the bald jokes.

If you ever wonder what you can do for a friend going through a difficult time, visit them. Your presence will communicate volumes and provide a welcome diversion and the encouragement they need. Don't worry about gifts or the right words to say. They don't matter all that much. A hug speaks volumes. Listening provides your ailing friend the opportunity to get a few things off their chest. The fact that you cared enough to go out of your way to visit says everything you need to say.

Chapter 12
Mid-Recovery

The plane keeps climbing through shifting winds and rough turbulence, but it's getting close to cruising altitude. The post-transplant cockpit crew is hard at work monitoring lab results, overseeing infusions, completing evaluations and checking medications. No new extraordinary complications have surfaced over the past few weeks, and my numbers are stable allowing for fewer hospital visits, less frequent infusions, and a longer leash.

We knew Dr. Kornblau would monitor my progress and make any necessary changes to the treatment process and anti-rejection drugs. We took it all in stride thankful that we didn't have to suffer through any more chemotherapy. The 91 treatments I had endured looked much better in the rear-view mirror. The new stem cells were doing their job and behaving nicely with their new neighbors. Another bone marrow biopsy showed that I was still in remission and my bone marrow was free of cancer. It looks like clear skies and smooth sailing over the horizon.

Not so fast. Without a chance to brace myself here comes some rough turbulence and another punch in the gut. Dr. Kornblau recommended follow up treatments of Vidaza, the chemotherapy drug I took before the transplant. Doc reminded us that 40% of transplant patients experienced a relapse and cited studies showing that we could lower that chance with a maintenance dose of Vidaza. Should any cancerous stem cells prove brave enough to make an appearance in my bone marrow, the Vidaza would kill them. It was hard to argue the point. The tough guy in me understood and was ready to roll. The ordinary guy in me was screaming in disbelief. After all I had been through, did I have to endure more chemotherapy? But, what could I do? If I turned down the chemo treatments and had a relapse, I would have a tough time living with that. Maybe it wouldn't last long. Maybe I'm in a state of panic over nothing. Maybe the treatments would be less painful. And, a good patient wants to do everything possible to ensure a successful recovery. Right?

I asked the question and readied myself for the answer.

"How much chemotherapy? How many cycles?" I asked.

The doctor's punch was well telegraphed. I could see the answer coming before I finished asking the question.

"Two years," Kornblau said. "We'll need to continue treatments up to your two-year transplant anniversary."

The oxygen mask just popped out of the overhead panel. Another two years of chemo? Seriously? That was a tough pill to swallow, and the big-league punch landed square in the gut.

I followed up with another probing question.

"How would we know if the chemotherapy was working?" I asked but I should have known better.

"We won't know," was the reply. "There is no way to track it. It just improves the odds."

We'll have no evidence that would confirm or deny the effectiveness of the chemotherapy. We would have to rely on those studies completed among other stem cell transplant survivors.

As usual, it was up to me. I had to make the decision. Move forward with the 24-month chemotherapy plan or opt out, spare myself the grief and take my chances.

What would you do?

A late friend, author, and former Navy Seal Richard "Mack" Machowicz would tell me to stack my advantages. Put as many assets on my side as possible before approaching any mission. Mack eventually lost his battle with brain cancer, but we had quite a few occasions to talk about the similarity of our struggles. His battle with stage four brain cancer was much more difficult than mine. I remember him getting mad when I stated, "Here we are, a couple of old guys circling the drain." He would never concede that point and fought like a warrior to the very end. For the most part, I tried to make it a point not to go around making Navy Seals mad.

I decided to put the lower dose chemo treatments in my stack of advantages. Mack would have made that an order. I made it a tribute to him.

Cindy and I dutifully reported to the 10th floor of MD Anderson for the first cycle of chemotherapy treatments. This time, cycles would be five days in length. I'll get one dose of Vidaza each day for five continuous days. After three weeks off, I'll be back for another cycle and more chemo. The Vidaza infusion took 15 minutes when administered through the PICC line still dangling from the inside of my right arm. When you add labs, prep time and waiting time it resulted in a two to a three-hour hospital visit. It was still an improvement over the previous seven-day cycles that took twice as long with three times the dosage. The first few treatments did not result in much discomfort. The fourth and fifth days were rough, and it took another day to rest and recover.

I responded well enough to the treatments and other tests required for a release from our nearby apartment. Another look at my lungs, eyes and internal organs confirmed my progress.

September 6, Day +84

Finally, the good news came, and it felt like a pardon from the governor. After a month in the hospital and the better part of two months in a furnished apartment within 15 minutes of the MD

Anderson emergency room, Cindy and I could finally go home. It's graduation day at MD Anderson, sort of. I had completed the required courses and physical challenges, and even though I was beaten up, scarred and worn out, I was now ready to take on the real world. I felt like I had completed BUDS training on my way to becoming a Navy Seal. Mack would have rolled his eyes at that analogy stating that I had no idea what I was talking about. I miss that guy.

One more visit with Karen and I was free to go. Karen, the survivorship nurse, is a specialist in the transition from hospital to home. She would help us tackle the brave new world as a transplant survivor. I hadn't allowed myself to claim that title. Survivor.

At MD Anderson a cancer survivor is defined as someone with a cancer diagnosis at the time of diagnosis and for the rest of their life.

"I like your numbers," Karen said looking over her glasses. "You're doing better than most patients at this phase."

I wanted to give Karen a fist bump but decided to stay more reserved and wait for the next shoe to drop.

"How would you rate your distress level?" she asked while she looked in my eyes to capture an honest answer. "Do you have any spiritual concerns?"

"Absolutely none," I replied quickly and returned her gaze. "I have no distress at all. I know where I am and have no concerns."

Karen studied my face for another second or two before accepting my answer and moving on.

The next shoe was more like a big boot. Karen slid a printed PowerPoint presentation across the table that included another massive list of do's and don'ts. Karen went through the list one slide at a time making us aware of the dangers once they unhooked our leash and we left the hospital safety net. The list pointed out the signs of potential complications and how to avoid picking up any new diseases. I had completed the Early Recovery stage and am now moving to Mid Recovery, a stage that could last up to two years.

We were shown the fashionable Medic Alert bracelets and encouraged to wear one at all times to identify me as a transplant survivor mandating irradiated blood products. Should I have an accident or required blood for some reason, it had to be irradiated. Regular blood would not mix with my new stem cells, and the result could be devastating.

Karen laid out some links to online resources available for information and assistance.

At this point, I'm ready for some good news. I needed some. I wanted to hear that I was making progress through the early stage of recovery. I was hoping the nurse would highlight how my blood counts had improved and described how the new stem cells were rebuilding my defenses. I was expecting to hear about all the new foods I could eat and the new freedoms I had earned. You would think I had learned to be more cautious in my optimism. Instead, the nurse delivered another punch in the gut. I still had no immune system. The Tacrolimus I was taking to minimize the rejection of the new stem cells worked to suppress it. The donor stem cells were being held at bay until my body was strong enough to handle them. I had to be babied for a few more months until they could reduce the Tacrolimus dosage and turn the donor stem cells loose to do their job.

The transplant also wiped out all of the vaccinations I had received as a child. Polio, tetanus, diphtheria. All of them. New injections would come in a couple of months when my system could handle it. But for now, I had no way to fight off the measles, mumps, whooping cough and other childhood diseases. That was a sobering thought, but it got my attention and emphasized the seriousness of this Mid Recovery stage. I had gone from the steady green light in my mind to a cautionary yellow light. I was listening more intently now to the nurse's instructions on how to survive this phase of my recovery.

While it feels like driving up to an overprotective school zone with yellow signs, flashing lights and volunteers with reflective vests carrying still more signs, some of the items on this bulky new list of do's and don'ts might be interesting or helpful to anyone wanting to avoid the flu or other common illnesses. What do you suppose is number one on the list to prevent infections?

And, the medical experts say...

(Can you hear the drum roll?)

Wash your hands! Use antibacterial soap and wash your hands before eating or handling any food. Don't even think about leaving a bathroom without a thorough washing. The hands should be scrubbed immediately upon returning home from any outing. If you want to take it a step further, anyone entering your home should wash their hands first. Everyone has to do that at my house.

I was never a fan of the surgical mask, but I had to wear one at all medical facilities, crowded areas and anytime strangers were within six feet during the cold or flu season. That's a lot more time behind the mask so I ordered a few nifty designer masks made of cotton that wouldn't irritate my face. The nurse made a strong point of avoiding anyone who had a cough, runny nose or any signs of illness.

Young children carry around all kinds of germs. Kids less than 12 are still to be avoided. That precaution pretty much eliminated the possibility of a visit to or from my four granddaughters. The chances of a visit at a time when none of them have a cough or a runny nose are slim. If they came within range, they would have to wash their hands and change clothes. I could see them running to Papa in slow motion with a big smile and extended arms intercepted by their mother and whisked off to the kitchen for a thorough scrubbing. That's a buzz kill.

Handling pets had a whole series of restrictions. I don't have any, so we skipped that part and moved on to the other no-nos like home remodeling, gardening, yard work and walking around in bare feet. If you want to avoid germs, stay out of the dirt. And, stay away from churches or other crowded places. There was that church taboo again. Dang.

The nurse spent a long time on food and beverage consumption. Foods must be thoroughly cooked. Never eat at a buffet and never order raw vegetables like salads in a restaurant or buy precut vegetables in a grocery store. Raw vegetables were okay at home if they are thoroughly washed and peeled. Other foods to be avoided are raw berries, nuts, honey and soft cheeses like Brie or feta.

The beverages to avoid include anything with alcohol in it. Alcohol doesn't mix with Tacrolimus or other medications. Thankfully, coffee is okay if I don't get carried away.

As the lecture went on, our attention waned, and our focus started to drift. We were given a document with all the notes we should have taken ourselves, so we didn't miss the sections on taking care of the skin, lungs, eyes, joints, and mouth.

I snapped back to full attention when the lecture topic shifted to the great outdoors. I was a guy who would spend most of my time outside if I could. But, not anymore. If I was brave enough to venture out of doors, I had to cover as much skin as possible with a hat, long sleeves, sunglasses, and sunscreen. So much for my tank tops and flip-flops. How do you walk around Margaritaville with all of that protection? How long would I have to wear all that stuff? Yes, I had to ask and, yes, you guessed the answer. Forever. Another punch in the gut. Right in the palm tree of my Hawaiian shirt. No worries, I saw this one coming. My skin would always be overly sensitive to the sun. The transplant put me at much higher risk of skin cancer or activation of GVHD of the skin. Do Hawaiian shirts come in long sleeves and UPF sun protection?

We proceeded to the topic of exercise, and the news got a little better. Walking and weight training help rebuild bone density. Running is fine if you can do it. I had a 10k to train for in six months, so I had to get going sometime soon. Balance exercise with periods of rest. Power naps are encouraged. Finally! A good excuse to catch a few winks in the middle of the day.

After a grueling hour and 45 minutes, Cindy and I left that class emotionally spent and thoroughly exhausted. Karen was a delightful lady and a solid professional that did a good job considering the subject matter she had to deliver. We were happy to be in the position to attend that meeting but were even happier it was over and were ready to head for home.

September 7, Day +85

We checked out of the medical center apartment the next day. After three months in the medical center, we packed the car and began the drive north to The Woodlands and home sweet home. This time for good.

It felt so good to unlock the front door and cross the threshold of our own home. Cindy and I felt like soldiers returning from an extended tour of duty. We had never been away from home for such a long period. Cindy made sure the home was spotless when we left. It remained spotless upon our return except for the dust that had settled in all the usual places. After a quick dusting and a once-over with the vacuum cleaner, we were ready to reintroduce ourselves to this familiar and comfortable space. It didn't take long to unpack and put our clothes in their proper places. Then, out the door for a walk along the Waterway. The air smelled like fall and the landscaping had been updated, but otherwise, the scenery hadn't changed. All the familiar points of interest were there. We had named one of the bridges over the Waterway "Prayer Bridge" because of its view of the skyline and the fact that we would stop for a brief prayer of thanks and guidance every time we crossed it. We stopped again on Prayer Bridge to give a special shout of praise and thank God for his deliverance. There is no place like home.

The return home provided a nice emotional lift. But physically, the nausea, weakness, indigestion, and fatigue continued along with dozens of other aggravating issues. Falling asleep was much easier in my own bed in my own home. Staying asleep was a different story. I'm confident that the chemotherapy reduced the size of my bladder by half along with my ability to control it. I awoke for three or four trips to the bathroom each night and tried to augment my broken sleep with a cat nap in the middle of the day.

I struggled with occasional dizziness that seemed to get worse by the week. Rising from a sitting position or standing after bending over was a sure invitation to a short dizzy spell. A few of those spells were frightening, and I had to reach for something to hold onto until the spinning slowed down.

It's amazing how the body will adapt. I got used to the myriad of ailments and dizziness and learned to get by with the new sleep pattern. I followed many of the no-no's I remembered from the big pre-release lecture. We continued to attend concerts at Cynthia Woods Mitchell Pavilion sitting in a sparse area of the lawn wearing a floppy hat and hiding behind my surgical mask. I reengaged with the men's group and enjoyed the weekly early morning gatherings keeping my distance from anyone with a cough or sniffle. We frequented the late afternoon church services each Sunday where we could find a few empty rows near the back door.

The surgical mask had found its place on my dresser along with my keys, money clip, and driver's license. They went into my pockets before I went anywhere. I looked funny at church, stores,

151

and restaurants but I got used to that too. I would be on the receiving end of looks and stares anytime we entered a store, restaurant or public place. The surgical mask and bald head gave away my cancer patient status and prompted some empathetic looks, a few smiles, and some unspoken well wishes. Or, people would feel uncomfortable and avoid eye contact altogether. I appreciated the empathetic looks and tried to return them with smiling eyes that communicated that I was doing fine. I understood the discomfort and avoidance. Some folks don't know what to say.

My favorite stares were from young children. Their inquisitive eyes looked right into mine maintaining contact as they pondered the possibilities. I always returned those looks with a smile and a wave. I would animate my eyes and wiggle my eyebrows to let them know their curiosity was welcome and to convey a sense of humor.

"Why is that man wearing a mask, Mommy?" kids would ask.

I would slow down my walk perking my ears in an attempt to hear the response. Some parents used it as a teachable moment. Most would give a short reply and continue their shopping.

I felt good enough to step up my exercise game a notch. Cindy accompanied me to the gym to lift some weights and resume my resistance training. She scrubbed all the equipment with some disinfecting wipes before I could touch any of it. What a shock. I could lift only a fraction of the weight I did before the transplant, and even that was a struggle. My new every other day routine with the wimpy weights wiped me out completely. It took a full day to recover.

Starting with a slow jog seemed like a good idea for cardiovascular exercise. I had the same result after a three-mile walk/jog around the Waterway. The short distance completely wiped me out. After two weightlifting sessions and as many walk/jog attempts I decided to put exercise on hold and stick to walking at a good pace. My 10k training would have to wait for a while.

It was hard to measure any improvement during the slow recovery, but I felt like I was moving forward. As the levels of anti-rejection drugs declined I would notice a little more energy and would become a little more active. We kept a close eye on any possible graft-versus-host disease, but no dangerous symptoms surfaced.

November 8, Day +147

Dr. Kornblau gave me a good once over during our monthly trip back to MD Anderson.

"Any pain?" he would ask. "Any falls in the last month?" "Any new problems or issues?"

I would confess to the bigger issues. The small ones I kept to myself hoping they would go away on their own. There were no big problems and no complaints to report this time.

"I think we can get rid of that thing," Doc said while he tapped on my PICC line. "Do you have any problem taking it out?"

Another milestone was at hand. A confident Dr. Kornblau didn't see any more intravenous medications or infusions in my immediate future and prescribed the removal of my PICC line.

"Are you kidding? Yank that sucker."

What a big positive, beautiful affirmative step towards recovery. Once detached from those lumens, I felt like a new man and a lot more normal. I didn't have to favor my right arm or avoid bumping into anything. Cindy didn't have to wrap it with Saran Wrap before each shower. There would be no more pain due to rolling over on it in the middle of the night. Best of all, there would be no visible physical evidence that I was, indeed, a cancer patient.

The PICC line had served as a constant reminder of all I had been through and the fact that another IV chemo treatment was right around the corner. Removing that PICC line was liberating in so many ways.

I sailed through the rest of my exam and qualified for the first series of immunizations to replace my childhood vaccinations. The first round began with five shots in the arm. I maintained my tough guy look, but those shots were painful! Cut your kids a little slack when they have to endure those injections. They may need to whine for a day or two like I did.

Life was returning to normal. Or, as normal as it could be. I frequently thought about what I had been through and how lucky I was to be in this phase of my recovery. It was too early to count any new chickens, but I was more and more hopeful for a few more years to do God's work. I thought less and less about my health issues and more and more about making the most of every day and every experience I was allowed to have. My focus on "surviving" each day gave way to a focus on "living" each day fully. I felt compelled to tell the story of God's deliverance every chance I had and to share the benefits of what I learned about living life one moment at a time despite bone marrow cancer or the difficult issues we face in this life. Why wait to share this story? Besides, God was about to provide a new stage and a much bigger audience.

Chapter 13

Resolutions

"There are two days in my calendar:
This day and that day." -- Martin Luther

God took away my tomorrow. But He left me with a much better today. While I have no assurance that I will see tomorrow, I will certainly have a productive, meaningful and joyful today. And, I wouldn't trade that for an ocean full of healthy tomorrows.

Jesus taught us to focus on today and not worry about tomorrow. "Tomorrow will bring its own worries," He said in the sixth chapter of Matthew. I am most grateful that He taught me that lesson even though it was a formidable lesson to learn. It took a fateful revelation and a rough and tumble fight with cancer for me to see the merit of those teachings. I hope that you can see the value in adjusting your perspective and know the joy in that teaching without having to endure a similar 2x4 to the side of the head.

Most likely, you are my brother or sister in Christ. You pray, read the Bible, attend church, follow God's commandments and have surrendered to a spirit-filled life. It's a great life, isn't it? There are no coincidences. Everything happens for a reason. There is an adventure around every corner. God opens doors and closes others. He leads us down paths we would never have considered on our own. Anything is possible. We are never alone. We are thankful and praise a God who is with us in every moment, loves us unconditionally and is continually working to transform our lives into the image of his Son. However, you most likely struggle with the teachings in Matthew 6, with the idea of living for today. We're not raised to think about letting go of tomorrow or letting go of our life and placing it in God's hands.

When you cast aside the worries of tomorrow, you find the pure joy in living for today. Unspeakable joy. You'll see firsthand the tremendous benefits in letting go. It's so hard to do, yet so rewarding if you can get there.

Let me go out on a limb and illustrate some examples by comparing a normal busy working family life with a life focused in the moment. In many ways, it may be a comparison of your life and my new life.

You'll probably get up in the morning, get ready and rush off to work. I'll rise a little earlier and take a few moments to enjoy the beauty of the sunrise. Then, get on about my day. I'll enjoy the luxury of a hot shower and linger a few extra minutes to allow that hot water to hit the top of my head and cascade down my shoulders while I contemplate the wonders that await today. At breakfast, I may get a few extra chews out of my toast and wonder why it tastes so good with strawberry jam.

You'll probably experience a lot of stress today and wonder if you'll get everything done. I'll wonder if I made the most of each project, meeting or conversation. I'll approach the day one event at a time. What is the real purpose of this meeting? Am I giving my full attention and everything I can contribute? Am I listening carefully to what my counterpart is saying? Am I missing an important message? Is there something else I can give? What else can I say to help that person, encourage that person or compliment that person? Usually, that is much more important than the actual project we may be trying to tackle. Am I making myself fully available at this moment to God and His good purpose?

You may hurry past a person in line at the grocery store. I'll consider that I may be in that line, on that day, at that moment to connect with that person in some way. Perhaps a simple smile.

Perhaps an extension of a little courtesy. Perhaps to offer some encouragement. Perhaps more. Is there something I am supposed to learn? Is there some wisdom in what they are saying to me? I don't want to miss the significance of that 'chance' encounter.

You may be irritated with a phone call rambling on too long. After all, there will be many more such calls, and you have many other things to do. For me, it may be the last time I speak to that person. I'll take my time with my friend and make sure they know how much I care about them. I'll ask if there is anything else going on that we should discuss. I'll take comfort from the time they take to listen to me. I'll appreciate their concern for me. Not in general but literally. Right now at this moment. I'll make sure that there is nothing left unsaid.

You may be a few minutes late to an appointment. I'll get there a few minutes early to collect my thoughts and to consider the pivotal aspects of that appointment. Why am I here? Why will they be here? How can we make the most of the next hour?

You may have weekly, monthly or annual goals. Maybe even a well-documented retirement plan. I have no goals or long-term objectives. My only concern is now. Will I make the most of the gift of this day? That's not to say that I don't have things on my calendar in the coming weeks or months. I do, and I hope many of those things come to pass, but I don't count on them. I look forward to them, but I don't hold on to them too tightly. And I certainly wouldn't put anything off today because of something else scheduled tomorrow.

At this moment, you may not be too concerned with the order of your priorities. There is plenty of time to work that out, right? If you are off a little today, no problem. You can rearrange things tomorrow. I don't have that issue. Without the burden of time, I continually and happily focus on what is most important. Now. Today. It is much easier to determine priorities and stick to them when you have no time limits, deadlines or target dates. Or, when you genuinely believe your time is short.

It may be one of those days. You may do what you need to do to get through it. After all, you can catch up tomorrow. Without the safety net of tomorrow, I have the motivation to push through whatever is holding me back and not let the day get by. There are no days to waste. This day could be one of but a few remaining. Maybe even the last. Who would want to spend their last day wishing it was over?

When your head hits the pillow at the end of the day, your unfinished projects may haunt you, and you'll wonder how you'll manage tomorrow's overbooked schedule. I'll give thanks for the day just completed and offer my vessel for His use tomorrow if it is His will. I'll enjoy a few extra moments of rest, quiet, peace and the warmth of nestling securely against the soft skin of my beautiful wife. I don't even assume I'll wake up in the morning and see another day. But, if it comes, tomorrow will be a great day. If not, I made the most of the day I had. Best of all, I look forward to that day, the glorious day of meeting Jesus, thanking Him, worshiping Him and spending eternity in that magnificent place he prepared for me.

Other authors may want to pace themselves and spread their creativity and perspective over several books or novels. This author only thinks of one book. This one. I better not leave anything on the table. I have to communicate everything I have to say and every aspect of this message in this one book. There may never be another. I'm not even guaranteed the time to finish it. Therefore, I better get everything I feel inspired to say on paper. Today.

You may wonder about your salvation. You have the luxury of time, or so you think. You may be up to your eyeballs in life on this earth today, but you are well intended. You'll make sure of your salvation soon. With all the time in the world, you may be putting off the aspect of working out your salvation or reducing it to one small step at a time. *"At least, I'm heading in the right direction,"* you might think. A person with no tomorrow or no time to wait clings to Jesus' words that today is the day of salvation. They take Paul's command seriously to work out our salvation with fear and trembling through his letter to the Philippians. They are working on it now. They make giant leaps rather than small steps because who knows how much time remains. And, wouldn't we want to face our Creator one step closer to the goal of Christlikeness? Isn't that more important than meeting a deadline at work?

Which life would you rather live? Which perspective would you rather have? I think that is what Jesus was trying to teach us. Taking the plunge, however, is hard to do. I'm here to tell you it is worth the effort and you'll love the benefits. If you can get across that bridge, there is true freedom and an incredible and rewarding life waiting for you on the other side.

Spoiler alert. It's almost impossible to get across that bridge by yourself. There are way too many distractions and too many things competing for your attention. God provides not only the bridge but the wisdom, yearning, focus, and power to get over the bridge. Don't try to do this yourself. Ask God for His guidance. Depend on His strength, not yours. He is waiting to hear from you with an outstretched hand and all the strength you need.

How does one with plenty of time suddenly start thinking that time is limited? From the perspective of someone pushed into that position, let me offer some suggestions.

Start with a simple first step. Put yourself in my shoes. What if you received the revelation? What if you heard the voice that I heard? What if your Creator told you He was calling you home soon? How would you react to that? Would you keep doing the same things the same way? Don't rush through that thought. Take a walk and contemplate that notion for a while. Ask God to speak to you about that perspective. Meditate on that idea. Let it simmer for a few days. Don't say, *"I couldn't imagine that."* Don't give yourself an excuse. Imagine it. Allow yourself to ponder your reaction to such a revelation.

Write down the things you would change if you heard the revelation. What would be at the top of your priority list? What would be the most important things to do? How would you spend your time? What things do you need to say? What amends do you have to make? What relationships do you need to reconcile? Would you feel differently? Would you think differently? How so?

When I received the revelation, I asked God for the time to get my affairs in order, finalize my mother's estate and get Cindy moved into a new home. What would you request? What three things would make up your "must do" list?

Consider that you have a short lifespan. You do. All of us do. You spend just a moment on this planet compared to the eternity that lies ahead. Yet, this moment seems so difficult to manage. There is so much urgency at this moment, this lifetime and so much that is visible and begging for attention. At the same time, eternity is an idea that seems to lurk at the end of a long road reached with steps taken tomorrow. It is so hard to look past what we see and what is staring us in the face and focus on what is unseen and awaits us in the next life.

The sobering truth is none of us have tomorrow. We only have today. God, in His infinite wisdom, didn't guarantee tomorrow. He gives us one day at a time and the free will to make decisions on how we will spend that day. He wants us to choose to live according to His will, depending on Him today knowing that He will take care of tomorrow. I can see Him rolling his eyes and shaking His head back and forth when we get all caught up in our plans for tomorrow.

Proverbs 16:9 tells us "In his heart, a man plans his course, but the Lord determines his steps." Our plans for tomorrow may not be worth much compared to the steps we take today. How many of our grand projects turn out as we imagined them anyway?

Make a list of the things that occupy most of your time now. Are those the most important things you can be doing? Make another list of the things that you would prioritize if you were being called home soon. Is the list different?

The next step is obvious. Shift your focus from the first list to the second list. Consider making the changes you contemplated when thinking through receiving a revelation.

This next question can be morbid, but it brings you face to face with a stark reality. When do you think you will die? Think about it. Then, give yourself an expiration date. Seriously. Given your current health, your lifestyle and your age, how long do you think you'll live? Subtract years if you are tightly wound, deal with a lot of stress or grapple with health problems. Add years if you are more easygoing and in good health. Be honest because this is important. Do you have the date? Not the year or the decade, but an exact date. Accuracy isn't the main issue. It's the consideration that there is a date. A date that you'll move from this life to the next life. Often our demise seems like a concept far in the distance. We don't want to think about it. We want to make it even more distant. What's essential is acceptance of the fact that such a date does exist and that it's not that far away.

Work backward from that date and place the most important things you'd like to do on a timeline between now and then. That exercise or thought process will move you from "someday" to "when." Let me take a bold step and suggest moving the critical things on your timeline closer to today. Closer to now. There is no guarantee of tomorrow, right?

When will you die? The correct answer is soon. God is calling you home. We can be sure about that. Our faith tells us that home is eternity with the Father and the Son and someday we'll get

161

the call. The time frame is soon. No matter how many years of life you can anticipate, compared to the thousands of years of history behind us and the infinite eternity ahead of us, the number of those years can only be described as a few. All of us are going home soon. Does embracing that fact change the way you look at your life today?

Here is another simple step in the form of another question. Would you trade places with me? Probably not. After all, I have a terminal illness. I'm dying. But, so are you. I have the luxury, the gift of knowing when. I know that my time is short. You think you have time to figure things out. You're healthy today. You are looking forward to tomorrow where you can put everything in its proper place. You're sure you wouldn't want to give up on all those plans you have.

Do you want to hear something surprising? I wouldn't trade, either. I wouldn't exchange the joy I experience today for the stresses that come from worrying about a lot of tomorrows. I wouldn't trade the joy in a few days that may include chemotherapy treatments or painful complications for a decade of good health that misses that joy because of a preoccupation with what happens down the road. I can say that with confidence. I've lived both lives. I've had both experiences. I can compare the two side by side, and there is no doubt in my mind. I choose to live in the moment. It was a tough journey, but now that I'm here, in the moment, I don't have any desire to go back.

Here's some good news. You don't have to choose. You're not limited to your current life or my life. You can have both. That's great news! You can have the joy and the rewards of living for the moment and squeezing the most out of each moment you have. And, you can live that way for many more years. Think of the possibilities and how much better life could be.

Use key events in your life to change your perspective. A friend of mine had a life-changing event while watching television a few years ago. The network news anchor reported on an airplane crash that took the life of John F. Kennedy Jr. That story packed a powerful punch. From my friend's point of view, John Jr. had everything. Good looks. A royal pedigree. Wealth. Excellent health. A great future with everything the world could offer. Then, in an instant, it was over. John Jr. went from everything to nothing. At least that's our perspective sitting where we are in the world. This tragic event cemented my friend's realization that life is short, much shorter than we think and gone in the blink of an eye. No one is immune.

I remember seeing my father flat on his back in the hospital recovering from a massive heart attack at the ripe old age of 55. He lay unconscious and lucky to be alive. A towel covered his midsection but he was unclothed from the waist up and the knees down. The harsh lighting gave his skin a yellow hue, and there were tubes connected to him in numerous places. It seemed like there were tubes everywhere. When I close my eyes today, I can still see that picture. My father was a good man well respected by the community and his family and friends. He was also a go-getter. A type A personality and always in motion. A driver. He seemed to manage it well, but he carried a lot of stress on his shoulders. The result of that fast-moving stressful lifestyle was right before my eyes. At that moment I decided to do things differently. That painful vision shocked me into choosing a different path. Nothing could be that important. I'd slow my life down and avoid some of the fried foods that Dad loved so much. As the decades passed, however, the memory of that scene faded or got pushed aside, and my life gradually increased in tempo.

What have you experienced in your life that had a similar impact? Have you forgotten about it? Has the memory faded over time? Think about those experiences. Bring them back and keep them close. They can help move you in the direction you want to go. They can be little 2x4's that work together to shorten your perception of the time you have remaining. Call them life lessons of which you will give much more emphasis. Don't let them fade or get pushed aside. Be thankful for them and keep them front and center. They can be useful to you.

Cindy and I talk fondly about our time and trials raising our two daughters. We took the job of parenting seriously, but the most memorable moments usually ended with belly laughs and a little embarrassment.

"If I knew they would grow up so fast and that our time would be so short, I would have spent more fun time with the kids and less time on housework and chores," Cindy stated in a recent stroll down memory lane.

I'll bet she'd like to get back the hours and hours she spent ironing perfect creases into the kid's clothes and my dress shirts. That's living for the moment in a nutshell. Treat each day as if time was short. Make the most of every moment. Forget the ironing and bake more cookies.

Think of a similar time in your life that was over before you knew it. Think what may be different if you knew that the time would go by so quickly. If only you knew then what you know now. Use that perspective to make the most of what you are doing today. You don't want to look back on these days and wish you would have done things differently.

I've made a habit of applying an "if/then" statement to most everything I do. If this thing I was doing was the last time I was going to do it, would I do it any differently? The 'if/then' statement is particularly effective with people. I'll often conclude a conversation with a statement like, "If this is the last time we have lunch, then I want you to know how much these lunches have meant to me. I enjoy your company and cherish every moment we had together." If it were someone special, I might take that a little further with a statement like, "If this is the last time we speak, then I want to make sure you know how much you mean to me. I love you and appreciate your friendship." Those statements were awkward in the beginning but quickly became natural and even expected. Who doesn't want to hear that they are loved and appreciated? They help me stay focused on what is most important and making sure I make the most out of what is happening right now.

Imagine traveling ahead in time to the end of your life. What happens then? Is there an afterlife? What do you believe about death, Heaven and hell? Are you doing anything in this life to prepare for the next life? Spend some time and do some homework on this topic. What you believe about what happens when you die will form the basis of what you do while you're alive. Many of us leave that all so important topic in the category of mysteries never to be solved. Perhaps the subject is too difficult to get your arms around. We'll have to find out when we get there. Knowing the short number of my years taught me that it's worth the contemplation time and the effort to come up with some concrete conclusions. Those conclusions can be uplifting and motivating. They are life-shaping conclusions. They result in great hope.

Talk to older people. Don't be afraid to bring up the subject. Chances are the shortness of days is at the forefront of their thoughts, and they would welcome the opportunity to talk about it, express their fears and share their perspective. It's one of my favorite subjects, and I would jump at the chance to convey my thoughts to a willing listener. Older folks are forced to come face to face with their mortality and deal with it whether they want to or not. Keep in mind, however, not all older folks want to talk about it. My mother remained in full denial until the day she died. If you happen across someone who is more open, the perspective that comes from those conversations could prove to be valuable to you and give them the chance to talk through it as well.

Consider why you are here. Why are you in this place at this time reading this book? Is there something else going on? Have you been led to this moment when, perhaps, you'd be open to the thought of making a significant leap in your thinking? Are you ready for such a step? I think that you might be.

This next exercise can be fun if you can get past its somber tone. Think of some typical things you experience on a day-to-day basis. Think of a phone call for example or a sunset, a concert, a football game or a church service. Now, think how that experience would change if you knew it was the last time you would experience it.

Would you hang up quickly if it were the last phone call you would make or receive?

How would the experience change at the last concert you would ever attend? Would you leave early? Would you go ahead and get the large popcorn at the concession stand? Would you complain because it was too crowded?

How about the last piece of pie? Would you wolf it down or take your time savoring every bite of that pumpkin goodness? Would you agree to that scoop of vanilla ice cream to make it ala mode?

Imagine that the beautiful sunset unfolding before your eyes is the last one you would ever see. Wouldn't you look a little more closely? Wouldn't you have a deeper appreciation of the splendor and the colors only God could create? Wouldn't you want to see it from the beginning to the last ray of light?

How would you treat the grandchildren if it were the last time you would see them? Would you be a little more patient? Would you go ahead and do one more pony ride? Would you give each one an additional monkey swing? Would you say no to any reasonable request?

I figured that each 10k I ran after I received the revelation could be my last. I ran those races differently. I didn't pace myself or slow down as soon as I usually would. I didn't keep anything in reserve. I ran the whole race with every bit of energy I had. Wouldn't you do the same?

One more. How about a church service? What if it were the last one you would attend? Would you open yourself up more? Would you sing the songs you knew? Would you be self-conscious about how loud you sang? Would you lift your arms if you felt like it? Would you pray more intently? What would you put in the collection plate? Would you rush out the door when the service was over?

I'd place a large wager that you would treat routine events differently if you knew it would be the last time you experienced them. You would get much more out of them. You would enjoy them much more. You would give more of yourself to them. You wouldn't hold back anything. Now you have a glimpse of how a life lived for today feels. You have a peek at the joy that emanates from those experiences if your perspective shifts a little. You have an idea of the joy you have been missing because you were looking ahead to the many competing entries on your crowded to-do list.

Focus more on now. This moment. We don't do that much. We tend to look ahead at what's down the road or around the next corner. We tend to look past now to the next thing on the to-do list or the next appointment on the calendar. As you sit, look up for a moment. Or, close your eyes and think about this moment. It is. Everything else either was or is yet to be. This moment is now. It's yours. It's yours to enjoy. To savor. To hold tight. What's so special about this moment? It's the beautiful things you can see. What are they? It's the warm emotions you can feel. What are they? It is all those things around you for which you can be grateful. What are those?

Cancel any thoughts about later when you can put this book down and take on another to-do list. Let go of that project with a tight deadline. Or, the chore you have to complete before your guests arrive. Squeeze every good thing out of this precious moment. Later, freeze the moment where you find yourself. At a concert, your favorite restaurant or walking to your next appointment, do the same thing. Look around you to see the beauty in this moment. Savor those things, say a prayer of gratitude, and hold them as long as you can then let them go. Lather, rinse, repeat. Make it a habit. Your joy isn't around the next corner. It's right here. Right now.

Finally, reread the gospels. This time pay close attention to Jesus' perspective and how He lived his life. Jesus models the perfect example of how God intended us to live our lives. Jesus not only contemplated the brevity of life but knew that His time was short. He knew He had an expiration date and exactly when it was. He knew that God was calling Him home. Soon. He seized every opportune moment to do what He came to earth to do. Teach, heal and preach the good news. He had no doubt why He was here and what He would accomplish. Not what He wanted to do. What He needed to do. What He was destined to do. What his Father sent Him to do.

Imagine the joy Jesus felt when He saw his faith rewarded. Imagine His delight when people experienced God's love through healing, when the lame walked and when the eyes of the blind opened. Not tomorrow but today. Jesus must have loved watching people flock to Him to hear His teaching and walk away praising God and starting new lives. He must have loved releasing His followers from their bonds and chains, forgiven and freed to pursue their relationship with the Father.

Jesus didn't waste one-minute building houses, planting fields or saving for retirement. He knew that God would provide. He knew that God was calling him home soon and placed His life securely in God's hands. He knew. He was happy. Extremely happy and He changed the world forever.

That's the wisdom of knowing the number of your days.

Chapter 14
Next Steps

By all accounts, my bone marrow cancer is in remission. On paper, I am still cancer free. There is every reason to believe I'll make it to that all-important two-year mark where medically, I can look forward to a normal life expectancy.

Maintenance chemotherapy treatments continue with their lingering side effects. I struggle with fatigue, weakness, dizziness, and nausea but I am adapting to those issues, and they are becoming less and less of a problem. I seem to gain a few taste buds here and there, and my appetite comes and goes. I'm skinny as a toothpick and must run around in the shower to get wet. I'm not yet regaining any weight. Monthly checkups and lab tests have all been positive and show I'm on the track of recovery.

Jim and Coleen have returned to their home in Florida where they are getting regular checkups and treatments at Moffitt Cancer Center. They return to MD Anderson quarterly for evaluation and follow up. They make sure they add an extra day or two to the visits to spend some time with Cindy and me. Jim has suffered through numerous complications in his post-transplant recovery including a blood clot in his left leg. Graft-versus-host disease bashed Jim in several areas. It dealt a knockout blow to his spleen and continued to pound away at his lower gastrointestinal tract. Through it all, Jim stands firm and continues his recovery little by little. We communicate regularly and get together when they return to Houston for their quarterly visits. I am grateful for these new friends and the positive impact they have had on our lives. They will be teammates forever.

Jacob is recovering in his Houston area home near the gulf. His kidneys are shot, he administers his own dialysis at home and struggles with lung problems. Even still, he maintains his upbeat approach to nearly everything. The transplant he received was successful and added a couple of good years to his life, but his prognosis is still grim. His Multiple Myeloma is in remission and most likely won't be the illness that claims his life. His other health struggles leave him with a life expectancy of about two years. Jacob has suffered through too many transplant complications, and his compromised immune system needs a periodic jump start with intravenous immunoglobulin or IVIG treatments. We get together when we can and talk about life within a short time frame, how it has changed us and what we're doing to make the most of the moments we have. There are not many people that are interested in that type of conversation, and I cherish every time we can get together. Jacob doesn't look back and wonder why he has been dealt such a lousy hand with his health. He doesn't look forward, either. He lives in the moment making the most of the time he has. Jacob is an inspiration and a joy to be around. When he can, he entertains a broad network of friends and crafts unique furniture and sculptures for his home near the waterfront.

My brother Mike is in complete remission. Like Jacob, he was diagnosed with Multiple Myeloma but in an earlier smoldering stage and received a stem cell transplant of his own at the University of Arkansas for Medical Sciences. The Myeloma Institute at UAMS is a leader in research and clinical care treating over 11,000 patients from all over the U.S. and 50 foreign countries. After completing the autologous transplant and follow up treatments, Mike is recovering at his home in Kansas. He resumed his teaching career and is reviewing several new career options that have come his way.

I try to lure him into retirement with stories of leisure and a vacation state of mind, but he will have none of it.

Dr. Steven Kornblau sees me every month and monitors my progress and the other patients lucky enough to be under his care. He continues to see patients and make the rounds while engaged in world-recognized research in the study of protein expression patterns in AML using reverse phase protein array technology. He founded and continues to head the MD Anderson Cancer Center Leukemia Sample Bank considered the most substantial tissue bank in the world. He travels extensively as a sought-after speaker and panelist for medical conferences around the world. He just wrapped up a nationwide research project that has identified some promising new protocols in the treatment of pediatric Acute Myeloid Leukemia. I am so thankful that he was assigned to lead my medical care.

Cindy continues to be a blessing to me and every person fortunate enough to cross her path. She held my hand, propped me up, carried me along and led us both through the biggest challenge of our lives. This incredible woman still sleeps with one eye open watching my every move, monitoring my breathing and checking my forehead for any sign of a fever. She tolerates my stubbornness, endures my complaining and is always there with unwavering support and the right amount of encouragement. Am I a lucky guy, or what?

Coleen and Judy continue in their roles as caregivers to Jim and Jacob. We couldn't have more appreciation or thank them enough for the many tasks, additional responsibilities and endless watchful hours they have contributed to our recovery. The role of caregiver is invaluable. Hospitals won't even consider a transplant unless a full-time caregiver is identified and near at hand. To Coleen, Judy, Cindy and all the caregivers everywhere, those of us who benefit so much from what you do thank you from the bottom of our hearts.

My life is different now. Different than two years ago. Different than six months ago. But, yours is too.

Two years ago, I was in great physical shape. I was running 25 to 30 miles a week, lifting weights every other day, and walking extensively. I retired early and had all the time in the world and the energy to pursue any path I chose.

One year ago, I was slowing down considerably. Chemotherapy treatments bogged me down for at least ten days each month. I could feel myself getting weaker with each treatment cycle. I knew I could pass away at any time with a few years of life left at the most.

Today, I even look different. When I look in the mirror, I see a different person. The hair is gone, and the face is longer with a few more wrinkles than I remembered. I appear to have aged about 10 years, and it shows in a shorter stride and muscles that won't go through their regular motions without a little warming up. I have to coddle an immune system in its infancy. I'm on the lookout for germs and viruses and avoid them at all cost. Internally, I am still healing from the harsh chemotherapy.

But my life expectancy has to be better. The doctors won't say, and I haven't pressed them for a new medical prognosis because I'm not so sure I want to know. I'm happy with the original three to five even though I'm chipping away at that a month at a time.

I am a bone marrow cancer survivor. I am a stem cell transplant survivor. I am alive two years after the revelation and a 1.1-year life expectancy. I am a lucky guy. In so many ways, the past two years have been the best years of my life.

The revelation turned my world upside down. It changed my thought process, my perspective and outlook on almost everything, for the better. I am so thankful for the revelation. It was a painful

2x4 that landed where it was supposed to striking the perfect spot. And, I continue to hold it close today. God will be calling me home soon.

I still don't know quite how to define "soon," and I no longer try. I don't dwell on that anymore or even think about it much. I relish waking up each morning and making the most out of each day God gives me.

Is there a future for me? I don't think about that much either. I do think about God choosing me for His revelation and what I am supposed to do with the changes that resulted from it. I don't want to squander that gift and sincerely desire that it achieve the intended result. When I do look forward, it's not in the direction of anything in this world. I look forward to eternity, and my next (and final) move to Heaven and the New Jerusalem.

There is no doubt in my mind that I am supposed to tell this story. God started something in my life. He planted a seed that continues to grow today, and there is no doubt that God will complete the good work He began if I submit to His will and follow his direction. I share my story and the joy of living day to day and moment to moment with everyone who will listen. God didn't give me this perspective intending for me to keep it to myself. He wants to continue to perfect this lifestyle in me and wants people to see a living breathing example of what He described in both the Old and New Testaments. He wants others to see my joy and hear the benefits of living life this way. God wants to bring this story to a new audience in a new way.

Am I the only one with this perspective or this story? Not hardly. But when would you say there are too many people telling this kind of story? Plus, each comes from a different angle. God led each of them to their place in a different way and gave each of them a different voice. I think He wants to keep telling us over and over again until we get the message.

As I approached the completion of this book, it was time to come clean with Cindy. I mean it this time! I can't kick the can any further down the road. There is no more road left. I wanted her input on the book and needed her to correct some critical details that I would surely misrepresent. She experienced every painful step with me and would have a valuable perspective and help add perceptive depth and nuance. I had to finally tell her about the revelation before she read about it in these pages.

December 6, Day +175

There wasn't a dramatic story behind the discussion we had while running errands on a typical fall day. We were sitting in the front seat of our car having a normal conversation. I didn't plan the confession. There was nothing set up in advance. I just couldn't talk myself out of telling her about the revelation any longer. As I opened my mouth to speak, the words came, and the tears flowed. She listened carefully with some tears of her own streaming through her stunned silence. She asked some questions but never challenged my assessment that the information would have been too much to handle. She didn't make me feel bad because I was so reluctant to break her heart more than it had already been broken. She didn't doubt the authenticity of my story or my interpretation. Instead, she thanked me for sparing her from wondering if each day in the hospital could be my last. She wondered that many times anyway.

Before I spilled the beans, Cindy felt like we had made it. We worked hard, endured a lot and made it through some difficult days. She understood the risks remaining and the high probability of a relapse. But for today, we beat cancer, and she was in full throttle victory mode. Thanks, Marc, for the cold blanket. Here comes another punch in the gut delivered by the person to whom she had devoted so much of her life. It was a return to the starting gate. She is still processing the revelation and what it means to us. Each day she feels a little more relief and a little more confident in a few more healthy years together yet still fearful that soon might be too soon. For now, she wishes for a bit more time together untethered to a nearby hospital hopeful that I live one day longer than she does.

From my point of view, it is such a blessing to finally have my best friend in on such an important part of my life and able to provide her wisdom and perspective. I was free of that ton of guilty bricks, that crushing weight of a secret I had carried too long.

We both agree there is a new mission ahead. We need to tell this story, and as I suspected all along, Cindy would support the effort and be there for every twist and turn no matter where it led or how long it would last.

With a stack of books under my arm and Cindy by my side, I'll be traveling from church to church and town to town wherever the Lord leads me. He'll open the doors and push me through them. He'll provide the story and tell it through me. God will pass some of this joy to others and show them what Jesus was talking about. I want Him to use me to convey why He would want us to live this way and the benefits of making that turn.

How long will this last? Not long. But God will fulfill the good work that He has started in me. That may be a week, a year or a decade. It doesn't matter. The only thing that matters is making the most of this moment and not missing this opportunity.

God may choose to extend my years as He did for King Hezekiah. The medical reports say that I could expect more years than the original prognosis I received a couple of years ago. If He gives me a few more years, I know He doesn't want me to slack off or allow my perspective to change. I don't want it to change. I don't want to go back to "someday" or "when I get around to it." I don't want to think long term. I don't want to make plans. I love today too much. I don't want to let go of now. I will hold tightly to the gift of living for the moment no matter how many moments He provides.

If you have received a dire prognosis, take heart. You're not finished yet. As long as you are breathing, God has a plan for you. All you have to do is ask, *"Lord, what would you have me do?"* And, I always like to add the word "today." *"Lord, what would you have me do today?"* He will provide the perspective, the strength and the wisdom you'll need to accomplish His will. He'll provide the peace and joy to make the most of your remaining days, weeks or years. He'll then welcome you to a new eternal home beyond your wildest dreams.

If you have gained some wisdom by knowing the number of your years, I'd like to hear from you. I'd love to hear how you arrived at that perspective and what it means to your life today. I'll bet it's fantastic. If you don't mind, I'll add your story to mine and tell it when I can. Who knows? Maybe I'll be around long enough to include some stories like yours in a follow-up book.

Whether you have a few days or a lifetime ahead of you, I hope you'll find your way to the joy that living for the moment provides. I hope you'll see the benefits and open your heart to Jesus' teaching. You won't want to go back or feel any differently. It feels that good.

God is calling you.

God is calling you *home*.

God is calling you home ***soon***. Maybe today. Maybe tomorrow. Maybe 20 years from now. Maybe in three to five years.

But, have no fear of your short-timer status. There is wisdom to be gained. The wisdom of knowing the number of your days.

Appendix A – Donor Letters

November 7, 2017

To: A Generous Stem Cell Donor

From: A Most Grateful Stem Cell Recipient

You have blessed me. Thank you.

Your generosity and compassion have given me the opportunity to extend my life and to live a better quality of life. Thank you.

Your stem cells arrived on the afternoon of June 14, 2017. They were infused into my body that evening by a top-notch team of exceptional medical professionals. Thank you.

Our tissues were a good match, and there was little rejection. Our blood types were even the same! Thank you.

The transplant was a struggle, but I had few options and my prognosis was grim. I had Myelodysplastic Syndrome, bone marrow cancer, and my God used those stem cells to heal my body. Thank you.

God used those stem cells to complete a good work He had started in me. He let me know that He had more plans for me and that He would extend my time on earth to complete them. Thank you.

Before the MDS diagnosis, I was a runner. I would pound out about 25 miles each week and run in various 10k, 10 mile and half marathon events. Not bad for a 60-year-old husband, father, and grandfather.

MDS slowed me down considerably. Perhaps it was the 91 chemotherapy treatments I endured prior to the stem cell transplant along with the symptoms of bone marrow cancer. A difficult year was capped with the news that the chemotherapy drugs were losing their effectiveness and there were no other options to consider. MDS has no cure. You fight as long and as hard as you can but the cancer eventually progresses and becomes fatal in 3-5 years. I was already one year into the fight and losing the battle.

It wasn't all bad, though. The year of fighting taught me many lessons about life, love and what's most important. When your time is short, your perspective changes dramatically. Silly arguments, grudges, personal gain or material acquisitions lose their appeal. Things of this world fade away. Things of the next world become prominent. Things like love, giving, receiving and improving relationships. Helping others becomes much more gratifying than helping yourself. You savor life's great pleasures like a warm breeze on your face, receiving a smile from a stranger or watching baby ducklings follow their mother across a still pond. What you can do to help brings much more joy than what you can do for fun. That's what God taught me through my struggle with MDS. We are to live our lives one day at a time. One moment at a time. Tomorrow will bring its own worries.

Now, things are different. Thanks to you, my outlook is brighter. Much brighter. I've survived the most difficult and physically grueling challenge of my life. Even today my body hurts. It struggles with weakness and nausea from the transplant and the side effects of a medicine cabinet full of medications. But, I'm happy to report that your healthy stem cells have replaced mine and today I am officially in remission. I am cancer free! Cancer free! The cancerous stem cells are gone. My doctor is weaning me off the anti-rejection medication. As a result, your immune system is becoming stronger and stronger in me. If I continue to heal over the next 18 months and weather any complications or a relapse, a normal life expectancy is possible. I have a chance. A real chance. And, I'm up for the fight. Thank you.

Rest assured. Even if I have all the time in the world, I'm not going to live my life that way. I choose to cling to the lessons I've been taught. Life is much better lived one day at a time enjoying every precious moment. You have given me many more of those moments. Know that I will relish every one. Thank you.

Please accept my sincere gratitude for your most generous gift. The gift of life to a complete stranger on the other side of the world.

If you are willing, I'd love to make the trip to see you someday and thank you properly in person.

With much love and respect,

A most appreciative
stem cell recipient
with much more
life to live!

28.02.2018

To: my stem call recipient

From: your donor

I am over the moon to hear that the transplant was a success and that you are now in remission. Thank you for reaching out to me and sharing so much that is personal to you.

The stem cell donation process is seamless, professional, swift and the experience is one of a prolonged but everyday, mundane procedure. Save for some bone pain and body aches as a consequence of the injections, it is also pain free. I have realised of course that, for the same reason that we have never communicated, this formality is all deliberate and it is to ensure that the donor never feels personally vested in the process. The closest comparison I can think of is making a charitable cash donation to an organisation that a close friend is raising money for. There is a small personal sacrifice involved, but every effort is made to desensitise the administration and make what you had always imagined to be deeply personal, *impersonal*.

Then I received your letter.

My wife and I cried. I never, ever cry but as I read it out loud I choked up. The faceless recipient of my stem cells was suddenly humanised. You have a family, are a loving father and grandfather and have endured the most horrific ordeal with cancer. And with any luck, and Lord knows you are due some, you can resume the same active life that you enjoyed before with a renewed sense of perspective. I honestly can't really do adequate justice with words to the emotions I felt absorbing that information for the first time. Satisfaction, joy, relief, fulfilment, happiness to name but a few.

Had I read your letter only 18 months ago however I am not as sure it would have had the same effect. I am sure I would have been elated that my stem cells had served their purpose but I don't know whether I would have identified with your story to the same degree.

My wife and I had our first child, a boy, in the recent past. He arrived at only 29.2 weeks so fully two and a half months early and at only 2.5 lbs. The next 52 days in hospital involved weeks in intensive care, high dependency and isolation wards as the amazing doctors and nurses worked tirelessly to first save his life, and then help him develop so we could finally take him home. It was a period that I will never forget, would never want to repeat but which I recognise as having shaped my lens on the world and which heightened my appreciation of life.

It is with that lens that I read your kind words. Though our experience pales in comparison to your own, I could appreciate the struggle you have endured and the life with your family that you, and they, must have been so desperate to prolong. Realising that my stem cells have enabled you to do just that is extraordinary and provides more gratification than you could imagine, and I needed none.

You should know that potentially more good might come of this. Your story has touched other people in my life and friends and family have already signed up for the donation process. It's such an easy, straightforward procedure and yet can provide the greatest gift. I feel incredibly privileged that my stem cells matched with your own and, of course, fervently hope that you remain healthy.

182

You are of course welcome to visit at any time, though I must confess that I am not sure how this can work whilst our correspondence remains anonymous.

With very best wishes for a healthy future,

Your stem cell donor

Appendix B - Scriptures on Living for Today

All verses ESV

Through all my medical trials, spending time in The Word was the best medicine. It provided encouragement, motivation, and assurance of God's healing power and boundless love for me. The Bible is our guidebook and applies to all of us in all our circumstances. No matter what we face, we'll find comfort and direction in God's Word. There are many scriptures related to health and healing and many on living our lives for today. Here are some of the scriptures that gave me comfort and direction along with a little commentary. They continue to remind me of my brief tenure on this earth and where my focus needs to be.

Psalm 90:12

"So teach us to number our days that we may get a heart of wisdom."

This verse was the inspiration for the book. Searching for the heart of wisdom gave meaning and purpose to both the revelation and the battle with bone marrow cancer. In this book, I hope to shed some light on this wisdom, to show how it applies to one person's life and declare its benefits to all. If you accept the fact that your days are numbered and how small that number is, a beautiful world unfolds and brings unspeakable joy to each day.

Psalm 39:4-6

"O Lord, make me know my end and what is the measure of my days; let me know how fleeting I am! Behold, you have made my days a few handbreadths, and my lifetime is as nothing before you. Surely all mankind stands as a mere breath! Surely a man goes about as a shadow! Surely for nothing, they are in turmoil; man heaps up wealth and does not know who will gather!"

David knew how short his life was. Even with all his worldly success and wealth, he knew it was fleeting and that he couldn't take any of that wealth with him. It was an excellent lesson for me. Accepting the fleeting nature of our lives helps us take ourselves much less seriously. It helps us focus on what is most important. Live for God, obey His commands and cling to the hope that is an eternal life well beyond this fleeting moment. Cherish your relationships and the opportunity to love your wife, hug your children and do something helpful for a neighbor. Don't put it off. Do it today.

Matthew 6:34

"Therefore do not be anxious about tomorrow, for tomorrow will be anxious for itself. Sufficient for the day is its own trouble."

I like the NIV version that states, "...tomorrow will worry about itself..."

Jesus was teaching about the futility of worrying about what we will eat or what we will wear or what will happen tomorrow. God will feed us. He knows our needs and will provide them. Jesus directed us to seek God's kingdom first, and all our needs would be met. Tomorrow will come if God wills it, but we shouldn't plan on it. Focus instead on what God wants us to do today. Right here. Right now. Rely on Him to meet your needs and direct your steps.

This command is one that most of us ignore. Yet, there is such a blessing in a life lived one moment at a time. I hope this book sheds some light on the many benefits that await if we can get there.

2 Corinthians 4:16-18

"So we do not lose heart. Though our outer self is wasting away, our inner self is being renewed day by day. For this light momentary affliction is preparing for us an eternal weight of glory beyond all comparison, as we look not to the things that are seen but to the things that are unseen. For the things that are seen are transient, but the things that are unseen are eternal."

The NIV version of this verse hung in a frame on my hospital room wall. I prayed for weeks looking for guidance on the one verse to take with me, and this is the one I was inspired to print and hang on the wall. I saw it every day in the hospital. It reminded me in the darkest most painful days that these afflictions were light in comparison to what lies ahead. These afflictions would last but a moment. When I couldn't see beyond my hospital bed surrounded by medical equipment, this verse transported me out of that room allowing me to concentrate on the unseen eternal bliss that awaited.

When I thought of Paul and all the afflictions he had endured, it made my sufferings pale in comparison. Still, Paul called those afflictions light and momentary. If he could do it, with God's help, I could do it. You can do it.

This verse was seen by visitors, doctors, medical staff and all who found themselves in my hospital room. I wanted it to convey a spirit of hope and encourage people to ask about how that verse applied to my situation. Who knows how God used that verse and the message he put in the hearts of those who saw it.

It now hangs in my home office as a reminder of how God saw me through those difficult days and the joy that awaits us.

Psalm 118:24

"This is the day that the Lord has made; let us rejoice and be glad in it."

When your days are few, this verse has even more meaning. I say this silently to myself every morning as I give thanks that God gave me another day. To let it go by without rejoicing and being glad would be a tremendous waste. To waste the day on anything other than God's good purpose would be unthinkable.

Proverbs 27:1

"Do not boast about tomorrow, for you do not know what a day may bring."

We as humans love to make plans and talk about the big projects we're working on and the career success that awaits around the corner. This verse is a warning to us and carries a lot of impact. It reminds us that we may not have tomorrow. Best to boast on the Lord and make the most of today.

James 4:13-14

"Come now, you who say, "Today or tomorrow we will go into such and such a town and spend a year there and trade and make a profit"— yet you do not know what tomorrow will bring. What is your life? For you are a mist that appears for a little time and then vanishes."

James relays Jesus' teaching in a little different way. He makes light of our silly plans relative to the mist that is our life. We put so much importance on planning, goals and long-term objectives and miss the real joy of today. There is unspeakable joy when we abide in Jesus and obey His commands. That joy is found in our focus on His commands today. It doesn't depend on how we plan or what we accomplish in the next month or so. Those plans usually interfere or keep us from experiencing that joy completely. We become focused on achieving the plans we made for ourselves rather than discovering the reason God created us in the first place.

Proverbs 16:9

"The heart of man plans his way, but the Lord establishes his steps."

So much for our plans. They aren't worth much. It's much better to submit to the Lord and let Him direct our steps today.

When we have big plans, we tend to change the focus of our prayers. We tend to ask God to help us achieve our plans rather than to submit to God's plans for us. If our plans come from God, if the Holy Spirit has given us a dream, that's a different story. But, if our plans are for earthly success, wealth and accomplishment, that may not line up with God's plan for us and provide major interference.

One step at a time directed by the Lord will get us where we should be going.

Psalm 89:47-48

"Remember how short my time is! For what vanity you have created all the children of man! What man can live and never see death? Who can deliver his soul from the power of Sheol?"

Here's another reminder of our short tenure on this earth and the certainty of our death. None of us has the power to cheat death or deliver our own souls. I find great comfort in looking beyond death to the eternal bliss that awaits us in the New Jerusalem. How about you?

Psalm 20:6-8

"Some trust in chariots and some in horses, but we trust in the name of the Lord our God. They collapse and fall, but we rise and stand upright."

We are tempted to put our trust in other men or women in positions of strength or power. We think if we have enough strength, money, weapons or tools, we can accomplish anything. In my case, the temptation was to trust the doctors or medical professionals that took such good care of me or the vast tools, medications, and equipment that were always near at hand. While I had a lot of confidence in the medical team at MD Anderson, my faith and trust were in the Lord. He alone would deliver me, if that was His will. He may use the medical team or the facility or the hands of a doctor to accomplish His good purpose. But if I were to survive, it was the Lord who would bring me through. I am so grateful He did.

Psalm 118:17

"I shall not die, but I shall live, and recount the deeds of the Lord."

I was most happy to cling to this verse after surviving the roughest days of the stem cell transplant. Again, God saw fit to give me another day. Not for my glory but His. He didn't save me so that I could make more money or win more awards; He allowed me to live to fulfill His purpose for me. To praise Him and glorify Him.

Proverbs 9:10-11

"The fear of the Lord is the beginning of wisdom, and the knowledge of the Holy One is insight. For by me your days will be multiplied, and years will be added to your life."

We can't extend our lives with exercise, stress reduction, a healthy lifestyle or building big walls around our houses. The Lord decides who lives and who dies. The Lord determines the number of our days. We should be thankful for every day that we have and spend it in reverence and awe of Almighty God. If we receive another day, do we allow God to use it? Are we submissive to His commands? Are we listening for His direction? Are we inquiring of Him every day?

2 Kings 20:1-7

"In those days Hezekiah became sick and was at the point of death. And Isaiah the prophet the son of Amoz came to him and said to him, "Thus says the Lord, 'Set your house in order, for you shall die; you shall not recover.'" Then Hezekiah turned his face to the wall and prayed to the Lord, saying, "Now, O Lord, please remember how I have walked before you in faithfulness and with a whole heart, and have done what is good in your sight." And Hezekiah wept bitterly. And before Isaiah had gone out of the middle court, the word of the Lord came to him: "Turn back and say to Hezekiah the leader of my people, Thus says the Lord, the God of David your father: I have heard your prayer; I have seen your tears. Behold, I will heal you. On the third day, you shall go up to the house of the Lord, and I will add fifteen years to your life. I will deliver you and this city out of the hand of the king of Assyria, and I will defend this city for my own sake and for my servant David's sake." And Isaiah said, "Bring a cake of figs. And let them take and lay it on the boil, that he may recover."

I love this story for obvious reasons. The chemotherapy treatments I received were becoming erratic. Typically, the chemotherapy drugs lose their effectiveness after about one year. Sure enough, at about that time, my blast count jumped significantly, and my blood counts were becoming less stable. When Dr. Kornblau proposed the stem cell transplant, I wondered if this "Hail Mary" could give me a few more years. But the revelation was clear. God said He was calling me home soon. Did God ever change his mind? Might he add a few years to my life? Was there any Biblical precedent for such a thing?

191

The story of Hezekiah seemed to be written for me. I was certainly no king. I didn't have Hezekiah's record of accomplishments, and I didn't have a battle looming with the king of Assyria. But God hears all of our prayers. God did add 15 years to Hezekiah's life after telling him to get his affairs in order. It could happen. I didn't interpret this verse as a promise, but it gave me hope. It told me to pray and pray hard. And to keep my options open.

Ecclesiastes 7:1-2

"A good name is better than precious ointment, and the day of death than the day of birth. It is better to go to the house of mourning than to go to the house of feasting, for this is the end of all mankind, and the living will lay it to heart."

You might have to have that 2x4 to the side of the head to take this verse to heart. It can be a little morbid to ponder but give it some thought in the context of living for today. How could the day of death be better than the day of birth? We need to look at it from God's perspective and not our own. The day of death for believers opens the door to the eternity for which we were created. We will then enjoy an eternity in the presence of God praising and worshiping Him in our new home, the new Jerusalem. The day of birth begins a life of struggle and trials. Short as it may be, life is tough. Birth is the first day of that short but difficult journey.

In the long run, which is better? To attend a feast or to mourn with those who have lost a loved one? In the world's view, a feast is a much happier place to be. In God's view, saying goodbye to a loved one reminds us of our mortality. The knowledge of that mortality keeps us focused on the importance of today knowing that our time is short, and we will have a similar fate. We shouldn't live for the next feast, but for the eternal life that lies ahead.

Just in case you need a few more reminders of the brevity of our lives, here are a few more verses to ponder.

Psalm 103:15-16

"As for man, his days are like grass; he flourishes like a flower of the field; for the wind passes over it, and it is gone, and its place knows it no more."

Psalm 144:4

"Man is like a breath; his days are like a passing shadow."

1 Chronicles 29:15

"For we are strangers before you and sojourners, as all our fathers were. Our days on the earth are like a shadow, and there is no abiding."

Job 14:1-2

"Man who is born of a woman is few of days and full of trouble. He comes out like a flower and withers; he flees like a shadow and continues not."

Isaiah 40:6-8

"A voice says, "Cry!" And I said, "What shall I cry?" All flesh is grass, and all its beauty is like the flower of the field. The grass withers, the flower fades when the breath of the Lord blows on it; surely the people are grass. The grass withers, the flower fades, but the word of our God will stand forever."

Appendix C - Be The Match Info

Every 10 minutes a person dies from some type of blood cancer. For many, a stem cell transplant could save their lives and extend the number of their years.

Many bone marrow and blood cancers are terminal. Chemotherapy treatments are intended to slow the progression of the disease and add a few years of quality life but are not a cure. The only potential cure is a stem cell transplant. The cancerous stem cells that have invaded the bone marrow are destroyed and replaced with healthy stem cells. It's a miraculous but risky and difficult process, and too often it's the only hope.

The stem cells needed to replace cancerous stem cells come from healthy people. They can't be manufactured or simulated. Stem cells have to be donated. The ideal donor is one related to the patient with a close tissue match. However, only 30% of transplant patients have such a donor. The other 70% must rely on unrelated people who volunteer to be donors. They rely on global registries like Be The Match.

Over the past 25 years, Be The Match, operated by the National Marrow Donor Program, has managed the largest and most diverse marrow and stem cell registry in the world. Be The Match and an anonymous donor literally saved my life and saves others every day.

In addition to the worldwide registry, Be The Match is engaged in research to find better matches, more timely transplants and more treatments targeting more blood diseases. The full story is available online at www.bethematch.org.

Over 13 million donors have registered worldwide. Thousands of patients are waiting for more donors due to the exact requirements for a tissue match. In all the United States not one person was a full match for me. The person with the closest tissue match was in Western Europe where the process of stem cell transplantation and the need for donors is much more widely known. My nurses told me that it is not uncommon to find a match in Europe much more quickly than in the U.S. because so many more people are registered. Awareness is growing in the U.S. as the process is having more and more success with more and more diseases.

The Stem Cell Transplant team at MD Anderson began the search for a donor the day I was diagnosed with Myelodysplastic Syndrome. If no related donors are a match, the team turns to the international registry. My siblings received their blood test kits, and out of 4 brothers and sisters, only 1 was a full match. My matching brother was happy to donate his stem cells and ready to go until he was diagnosed with a disqualifying blood cancer of his own called Multiple Myeloma. Lucky for me a donor was found matching 13 of 14 key HLA (Human leukocyte antigen) markers. Ten of those markers are considered a high priority and the donor matched all 10. The immune system uses HLA markers to recognize which cells belong in the body and which do not. The closer the HLA match, the fewer complications from the stem cell transplant. The donor selected for me was a 33-year-old male who had registered in Western Europe.

Registration is not that complicated. A phone call to 1-800-marrow2 or registering online at www.bethematch.org gets the process going. You'll receive a swab kit in the mail with directions on how to swab your cheek and return the saliva sample. It's that simple. Once registered, researchers will match your tissue with potential recipients. It may take a while to find a match but be ready to donate.

If you are selected, you'll donate cells with a process called Apheresis. You'll get some injections of Neupogen for several days before the Apheresis that cause the bone marrow to make extra stem cells and release them into the bloodstream. I've had many Neupogen shots myself administered with small needles usually in a fatty part of the stomach. I can tell you that they are not too painful. A nurse pinches about an inch of skin then skillfully injects the Neupogen.

Once the stem cells are ready for harvesting, nurses connect you to a machine that draws blood from one arm, extracts the stem cells it needs then returns the blood to the other arm. The procedure takes up to four hours. The Apheresis process may have to be repeated two or three more times to get the required number of stem cells. I've had peripheral lines placed in my arms 91 times for the infusion of chemotherapy treatments. Speaking from experience, that's not so bad either. It's no more painful than a pinch.

The Neupogen shots can cause some headaches and body aches, but they go away shortly after the donation.

The harvested stem cells are usually processed and frozen (if necessary) then shipped to the hospital for infusion in the patient. The stem cells I received were donated in one day, flown to MD Anderson hospital and infused the next day.

All I know about the generous donor is that he is a 33-year-old male from Western Europe. The identity of the donor and recipient are kept anonymous for two years. If both parties agree, they can share identities after the waiting period. I wrote my donor a letter upon receipt of his stem cells (located as an appendix in this book) and look forward to thanking him personally when I hit the two-year mark.

The idea that a person in a foreign country would donate stem cells to save or extend the life of a person they don't even know half a world away still blows me away. I hope you'll consider registering at Be The Match and giving some life-saving healthy stem cells to someone that needs them. You might blow them away.

Be The Match

1-800-marrow2

www.bethematch.org

Appendix D – Critical Decisions

Cancer patients and anyone going through a serious trial in their life faces many critical decisions. Many of those decisions fall in the life or death category. They can determine the quality of life or the timeliness of death. Patients can open themselves to the assistance and support of others or try to face situations alone. Below, I've detailed a few of the critical decisions in *The Time Of My Life*. Would you have made a similar decision? Are you facing similar situations in your own life? How will you approach these inevitable forks in the road?

Continue running or stop?

Chapter 1: Revelation.

During a routine run around the neighborhood, the notion to stop running came upon me. It was an urge to stop running and listen. I don't know how many times in my life I have heard a similar message or felt a similar urge. Usually, they are dismissed as random thoughts in the name of a discipline to complete the task I had set out for myself. I almost did that during this run. I was feeling good and had a great pace going. I would have been happy about my finishing time. The urge persisted, however, and I finally decided to indulge it and stop. That stop changed my life. The fateful revelation came during that stop. Had I not plopped down on that park bench, I may have never received God's impactful message.

How many times have you dismissed the urge to do something different? To change your path, say something to a friend, run a different way or stop what you're doing? God speaks softly to us guiding our steps. So softly we sometimes can't hear it. The noise around us drowns it out. Or, maybe we're not listening. Ask God to open your heart and to help you discern between random thoughts and his gentle voice. Imagine what you might be missing!

Accept one of the treatment options at the first clinic or get a second opinion?

Chapter 3: Diagnosis.

I remember my conversation with Cindy walking out the front doors of the clinic. We had no idea what to do or how to proceed. We had to process a cancer diagnosis and determine if we wanted to move forward with that doctor and that facility. That critical decision was the first to fall in the life or death category. Should we stick with the familiar clinic and the doctors who found the cancer? Or, take advantage of the world-renowned cancer experts a few miles down the road.

This decision came quickly to Cindy. She was all in for a second opinion. I was waiting for a professional referral before moving forward but she thought I was wasting valuable time. Every minute that passed without a phone call from me and an appointment at MD Anderson was a minute that cancer could be growing. In her mind, I shouldn't wait another second. I should get on the phone that minute.

Once I made the initial phone call, the wheels went into motion quickly. The admissions department at MD Anderson acted swiftly and made things easy for me. I provided some necessary information and confirmation of my previous diagnosis, and we were off to the races.

When people seek the advice of a survivor, the first thing I suggest is a second opinion. An additional round of testing is no fun, but the confidence that comes from the confirmation is worth its weight in gold. There will be times when treatments cause extreme suffering and strong second thoughts. You'll question your decisions many times. That extra layer of confidence will help you pull through those difficult times.

Move forward with the MDA treatment plan?

Chapter 3: Diagnosis.

While I had a lot of confidence in Dr. Kornblau and that extra layer of assurance from the second opinion, the decision to move forward with the recommended treatment plan was not automatic. It was a life-changing decision. We would be making the transition from everyday folks to cancer patients and a dramatic lifestyle change. We would have to build our lives around doctor appointments and chemotherapy treatments. I would have to endure all those nasty side effects and the wear and tear on my aging body. If God was calling me home soon, why go through all that pain and suffering? Why not ride out the rest of my days and take life one day at a time?

We took our time with this one and put some serious prayer time behind our decision. We put it completely in God's hands and trusted Him to point the way forward. My biggest regret is not doing the same thing for every one of our choices. Some we made quickly. Some decisions we made instinctively. We depended on our human experience and usual decision-making processes for the desired outcome. As children of the Most High God, He wants us to bring these decisions to Him. All the decisions. Every one. We are to trust that He knows what is best for us, sees the past and future and has the perspective we will never have. The decision to trust Him with our decisions was the best decision we ever made.

God directed us to the treatment plan. He taught us many things about ourselves. He brought us together with people we would have never otherwise met. Our Father opened our hearts to the plight of others. He put us in a position to be helpful to other struggling cancer patients. God wanted a little more of His light to shine at MD Anderson through us. We are so thankful He used our vessels to accomplish that task.

Endure the transplant or stay the course?

Chapter 8: Preparation for Transplant.

There was no doubt in my mind that this decision was well beyond my ability to reason. I had much too little knowledge about stem cell transplants and no idea what it would do to me. Once I checked in the hospital, I had no clue how I would check out or even if I would check out.

The chemotherapy treatments I had been taking were losing their effectiveness. If I didn't endure the transplant, my cancer would most likely progress into Acute Myeloid Leukemia and cause my inevitable death. But transplants only work half the time, and there is a good chance I may endure all that grief for nothing. I may not even survive the transplant.

It was not an easy decision and I didn't even try to make it. I admit it was easy to accept my position of ignorance and leave the decision to the Creator who knew exactly what to do. There was no question I was way out of my league. When you have no answer, it is easy to depend on the direction of a loving Father. It was easy to go to Him and ask the direct question, "What would you have me do?"

What was my Father's advice? He said it didn't matter. He was bigger than cancer and bigger than transplants. He put the decision back in my lap. What would I do with that? What was I supposed to learn from that? Do I take the spiritual path and forgo the transplant placing cancer in His hands only? Do I take advantage of the best cancer care in the world just a few miles down the road? I may have felt guilty about accepting the medical treatments if the Lord would not have said that it didn't matter.

I decided to move forward with the transplant with one cautious eye on the possibility I was heading down the wrong path. I kept listening for the conviction of the Holy Spirit that I would feel when it was time to shift gears or correct some negative behavior. I never heard or felt that conviction as the transplant process moved forward.

With 20/20 hindsight, I do not doubt that I was meant to go through the transplant and have the experiences that went with it. I was meant to meet the people that crossed my path and bring some spiritual light into a place that needed it badly. I was meant to survive long enough to tell the story.

What kind of pain relief?

Chapter 10: Post-Transplant

Out of all the experiences I had in and out of the hospital, this was the most undeniable test of my faith. While I was struggling with the pain of excruciating headaches, God reminded me of a past promise made during previous chemotherapy treatments. He would relieve the headache pain if I put my trust in Him. I was to endure the other symptoms and side effects, but the headaches were His.

The decision was clear. The fork in the road was plain to see. Take medication to ease the pain or trust God for relief. Take the medical path or take the spiritual path. Take the sure bet of modern science or take a leap of faith. Take the road most socially acceptable or stand firm in a decision that many might question. Use your head or use your heart.

The questions were right before me. What do you believe? What do you *really* believe? Does God know of the struggle? Is He watching now? Does he heal people like me? Was this an actual reminder from God or was it a delusional rose-colored thought? How much faith do I have? How much trust am I willing to apply? How dependent am I willing to be?

I had one advantage. God had relieved my pain before. He asked me to give him the headaches in the past, and He fulfilled His promise. While the headaches I felt during the stem cell transplant were many times stronger and more painful, they certainly hadn't grown big enough to overpower the Creator of the universe. Trusting him with an even more crippling pain wasn't that much of a stretch.

The pain took me to a new level where I stood at the brink. I couldn't bear it for another minute let alone patiently wait for a miracle. I had to make a decision quickly.

All of us face those decisions at various times in various circumstances. We routinely meet little tests of faith and occasionally, major tests of faith. In my experience, passing smaller tests resulted in facing larger tests. Those tests continue to escalate until we face the biggest test of all. Are you willing to go all in? Trust God with everything in your life? Fully submit to Him in every circumstance? Leave the consequences to Him? Obey every command? Follow Jesus no matter what the cost? In my experience, the joy felt upon passing the tests and obeying the commands grew with the size of the test. The bigger the test, the greater the joy. The more fully you submit, the more joy you experience.

Can you imagine the feeling I had when the pain subsided? That feeling of gratitude, appreciation and utter joy? Can you imagine being free of that level of suffering with no drugs at all knowing that the relief came from God? Putting faith and trust in God is always the right thing to do.

Stay an additional ten days in the hospital or leave with traces of the bacteria?

Chapter 11: Early Recovery

After surviving a stem cell transplant and spending a month in a sterile hospital room, I was ready for some fresh air, sun on my face and a change of scenery. My body was gaining strength, and I was avoiding some of the typical complications from the stem cell transplant. The doctors allowed me to leave the floor and do some walking around the hospital. That small taste of freedom created a desire for more, and I was nearing the time when most patients are released. I could taste it. I was ready to go.

Doctors posted a conditional release date, and the finish line was now in clear view. All I needed was a little luck and no unexpected problems.

The only issue standing in my way was the "Capno-cytophaga Sputigena" bacteria that somehow found its way into my blood stream. The infectious disease team wouldn't clear me if any evidence of the bacteria remained in my system. I couldn't feel it. The bacteria didn't cause any pain or discomfort. It was just there. A generic antibiotic was prescribed to kill the bacteria while the labs worked on a custom version that would be more effective and deliver the final knockout blow. But, no luck after a week or so of testing.

The day before my scheduled release date, the infectious disease specialist gave me an update and a decision to make. The custom antibiotic could take another week to develop and another couple of days to eradicate the bacteria. They recommended staying in the hospital until no trace of the bacteria remained, but the decision was up to me. They would release me with the generic antibiotic with 80% certainty that the progress over the last two weeks would continue. Or, I could stay in the safer hospital environment until blood tests indicated the bacteria had been eradicated.

What would you do?

The answer came quickly even before I had the chance to get on my knees and make a formal inquiry of the Lord. I knew I had to stay. Cindy took a strong stand firmly encamped with the doctors stating that we had spent four weeks in the hospital and another week or two wouldn't be the end of the world. There had been too much sacrifice and too much effort made by too many people to walk out the door and roll the dice. We would stay, honor the medical teams' hard work and leave with a completely clean bill of health.

I could see the doctor's eyes light up and detected some relief on his face when I told him we would stay. I felt God's peace secure in the knowledge that He was leading us in this direction.

Was this another little test? Was I to indulge my impulses and immediate desires or demonstrate some self-control, the kind provided by the Holy Spirit? This decision eclipsed saying no to a few tasty calories or holding your tongue in a heated conversation. This decision required a whole new level of patience.

The next day, we got the news that the folks in the lab identified another generic antibiotic that would do a better job of attacking the pesky bacteria. The doctor stated that he was 95% sure it would complete the task and had no problem releasing us.

Was this a coincidence? Did I get a break? Was it a simple stroke of good luck?

Should I agree to maintenance chemo treatments?

Chapter 12: Mid-Recovery

I was enjoying time outside the hospital. Even though I wasn't home, I had some freedom. I could walk the aisles of the grocery store or stroll through Hermann Park. I could ride in the car and take in the familiar sites of the Medical Center. I could see for miles well beyond the medical buildings that surrounded the hospital.

The appointments were getting fewer and lab results stable. I was making progress.

I could continue making progress and lower the chances for a relapse with a regimen of follow up chemotherapy. Studies showed that a monthly dose of Azacitidine would minimize the growth of any cancerous stem cells that may find their way into my bone marrow. There was a 40% chance of those stem cells returning, and the percentage tended to decrease among those taking the chemotherapy. The treatments were recommended, but there would be no solid evidence if they had any impact at all on the cancerous stem cells.

All you have to do is take ten shots in the stomach each month. Two shots per day for five continuous days every four weeks. That means go to the hospital, check in, wait for a room, take a nausea medication, wait for the labs to mix the drug then get the two shots. It's a good two hours start to finish. Five days a month. Every month until my two-year transplant anniversary. That's a total of 220 shots in the stomach but who's counting? Will it work and keep any returning cancerous stem cells at bay? You'll never know.

It's not an easy decision. What would you do?

I used my head on this one instead of my heart. I confess to making this decision on my own. I went with the odds. As I gazed down the 22-month road, I could see an outcome where I had a relapse, and the cancer cells returned. If I had shunned the chemotherapy treatments and didn't do everything I could do as a patient to stop cancer's return, I couldn't forgive myself. I wouldn't be able to look into the eyes of those I love knowing that a dismal outcome might have been avoided. I owed it to them. And, I owed it to myself to do everything I could do to ensure the best possible result.

Should I have placed my faith squarely into the hands of the God who heals? Should I have trusted that He would protect me from a relapse? I'm not so sure I did the right thing. I'm not so sure that a bold step of faith might have been the better way to go. I will always wonder.

Should I tell Cindy about the revelation?

Every chapter.

I asked myself that question every day for a little over two years. Should I tell Cindy about the revelation? How would she react? Should I share this news or shoulder the concern on my own? Would full disclosure serve any purpose? How could I keep this to myself?

Cindy has an abundance of great qualities. She is kind, generous, funny, loving and the best companion a person could hope for. She is also a worrier. The revelation would have been a heavy load for her to carry. She would worry about it constantly. Anyone would, but she would take it a few steps further. It would keep her awake at night. Every night.

Cindy is also a strong woman of faith. I have seen her rise to every occasion no matter how difficult and she has shouldered crippling responsibilities over her lifetime. She is no weakling. No wallflower. Everything I believed and had witnessed should tell me she could take it. She could handle the news. There would be no better confidant. There would be no human being with more wisdom to impart or more perspective to provide. No one who would be more supportive.

Didn't she deserve my respect? Wasn't she owed the truth? The good, bad or ugly truth no matter what?

I chickened out. I kept myself from the uncomfortable position of trying to explain it. I went with the excuse of protecting my wife from many sleepless nights, endless worry and unwieldy stress. I didn't have faith in her inner strength and her ability to process the revelation. I didn't have faith that God would steer her through this valley, comfort her and provide the same peace that He provided me. Why?

That decision haunts me still today. While things worked out okay and Cindy forgave my selfishness, I'm sure this journey would have been much easier if she were in on the revelation. She endured every other challenge and every other punch in the gut. She would have done the same with the revelation.

If only I would have submitted to the guidance and direction of my heavenly Father. He knew. He saw both of us for who we were. He knew our hearts. He knew our weaknesses and the comforting power of His strength. He saw far beyond my feebleness and shortcomings. He sees what can and will be. I can only see what might be. Why depend on myself and my limitations for something so important?

Any decision should be presented to our God ahead of time. He is there. He is listening. He wants us to come to him with every option and every circumstance without restriction or limitation. He can handle all my issues along with every one of yours and every other person on this planet and beyond. Why put limits on God? Why ask ourselves if our problems are too small, too trivial or not important enough for His consideration? He has been there with comfort and strength at every bend and turn. He has fulfilled every promise. He has forgiven every misstep. Why not lean fully into that kind of love?

What should you do?

About The Author

Marc McCoy is a writer, speaker and workshop facilitator who challenges audiences all over America to make the most of every living moment.

His speeches and workshops are filled with humor, optimism and practical information on how to face life's most difficult questions. He offers constructive solutions to the problems and obstacles that keep most people from having the time of their lives. Attendees come away with new perspectives, new priorities and a renewed sense of hope and purpose.

Attendees dealing with a cancer diagnosis and difficult treatments will smile when they recognize and share the challenges and absurdities they face along a most painful journey. They will be challenged to accept a dire prognosis. They will see a path through their difficulties to a beautiful new world and appreciate the rare opportunity to see it.

Marc lives in The Woodlands, Texas with his wife, Cindy. He learns, teaches and worships at The Woodlands United Methodist Church.

Here's how to reach Marc McCoy:

marc@mccoybooks.com

@marcmccoy325

www.mccoybooks.com

Need an extra copy of *The TIME of my LIFE* to pass along to a loved one?

Visit www.amazon.com